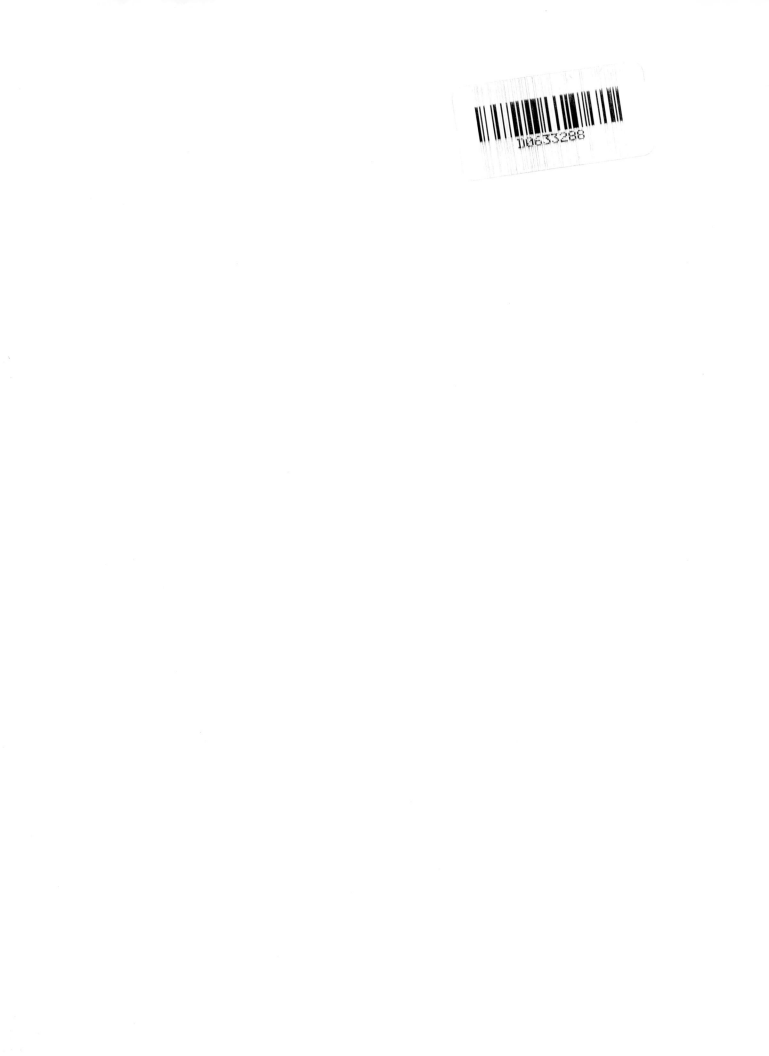

FOURTH EDITION

ACSM's Health/Fitness Facility Standards and Guidelines

American College of Sports Medicine

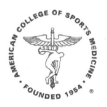

Senior Editors

Stephen J. Tharrett, MS, ACSM Program Director®
Club Industry Consulting, Dallas, TX

James A. Peterson, PhD, FACSM
Healthy Learning, Monterey, CA

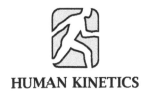

HUMAN KINETICS

Library of Congress Cataloging-in-Publication Data

American College of Sports Medicine.
  ACSM's health/fitness facility standards and guidelines / American College of Sports Medicine ; senior editors, Stephen J. Tharrett, James A. Peterson. -- 4th ed.
      p. ; cm.
  Health/fitness facility standards and guidelines
  Includes bibliographical references and index.
  ISBN-13: 978-0-7360-9600-3 (hard cover)
  ISBN-10: 0-7360-9600-0 (hard cover)
1. Physical fitness centers--Standards--United States. 2. American College of Sports Medicine. I. Tharrett, Stephen J., 1953- II. Peterson, James A., 1943- III. Title. IV. Title: Health/fitness facility standards and guidelines.
  [DNLM: 1. Physical Education and Training--standards--United States--Guideline. 2. Health Facilities, Proprietary--standards--United States--Guideline. 3. Physical Fitness--United States--Guideline. QT 255]
  GV429.A45 2011
  613.7'1--dc22
                                      2011004063
ISBN: 978-0-7360-9600-3

The web addresses cited in this text were current as of January 16, 2012, unless otherwise noted.

Acquisitions Editor: Amy N. Tocco; **Managing Editor:** Amy Stahl; **Assistant Editor:** Rachel Brito; **Copyeditor:** Patricia L. MacDonald; **Indexer:** Betty Frizzéll; **Permission Manager:** Dalene Reeder; **Graphic Designer:** Robert Reuther; **Graphic Artists:** Robert Reuther and Kim McFarland; **Cover Designer:** Keith Blomberg; **Art Manager:** Kelly Hendren; **Associate Art Manager:** Alan L. Wilborn; **Illustrations:** © Human Kinetics; **Printer:** Total Printing Systems

ACSM Publications Committee Chair: Walter R. Thompson, PhD, FACSM; **ACSM Group Publisher:** Kerry O'Rourke

Human Kinetics books are available at special discounts for bulk purchase. Special editions or book excerpts can also be created to specification. For details, contact the Special Sales Manager at Human Kinetics.

Printed in the United States of America.   10 9 8 7 6 5

The paper in this book is certified under a sustainable forestry program.

Human Kinetics
Web site: www.HumanKinetics.com

United States: Human Kinetics
P.O. Box 5076
Champaign, IL 61825-5076
800-747-4457
e-mail: humank@hkusa.com

Canada: Human Kinetics
475 Devonshire Road, Unit 100
Windsor, ON N8Y 2L5
800-465-7301 (in Canada only)
e-mail: info@hkcanada.com

Europe: Human Kinetics
107 Bradford Road
Stanningley
Leeds LS28 6AT, United Kingdom
+44 (0)113 255 5665
e-mail: hk@hkeurope.com

Australia: Human Kinetics
57A Price Avenue
Lower Mitcham, South Australia 5062
08 8372 0999
e-mail: info@hkaustralia.com

New Zealand: Human Kinetics
P.O. Box 80
Mitcham Shopping Centre, South Australia 5062
0800 222 062
e-mail: info@hknewzealand.com

E5198

Contents

Senior Editors and Associate Editors

SENIOR EDITORS

Stephen J. Tharrett, MS
Club Industry Consulting
Dallas, Texas
Formerly with Russian Fitness Group
Moscow, Russia

James A. Peterson, PhD
Healthy Learning
Monterey, California

ASSOCIATE EDITORS

Paul Eigenmann, MS
QualiCert
St. Gallen, Switzerland

Hervey Lavoie
Ohlson Lavoie Corporation
Denver, Colorado

Frank Napolitano
GlobalFit
Philadelphia, Pennsylvania

Walter R. Thompson, PhD
Georgia State University
Atlanta, Georgia

Cary H. Wing, EdD
Medical Fitness Consultant
Formerly with Medical Fitness Association
Richmond, Virginia

Preface

The benefits of engaging in a physically active lifestyle are both numerous and well documented. To achieve these benefits in a safe and efficient manner, individuals should adhere to a few well-defined training principles and guidelines while exercising. Furthermore, it can be extremely useful for an individual to have access to resources (e.g., fitness equipment, professional staff, and well-designed exercise programs) that can help ensure a positive exercise experience.

Not surprisingly, millions of people have chosen to join health/fitness facilities (such as YMCAs, Jewish community centers, commercial health/fitness clubs, public recreation centers, medical fitness centers, and corporate fitness centers) that can provide them with the tools and exercise environment that they perceive they need to be physically active. All factors considered, the better managed these facilities are, the more likely they will be to provide their users with exercise experiences that are safe, time efficient, and effective.

The focus of the efforts surrounding the development of the fourth edition of *ACSM's Health/Fitness Facility Standards and Guidelines* has been to establish a blueprint that specifies what health/fitness facilities must do to maintain the standard of care that they offer their members and users, and what health/fitness facilities should provide in order to enhance the exercise experience that members and users can achieve by taking advantage of the activities and programs offered by a particular facility. Before the publication of the four editions of this landmark text, no such blueprint existed. Appendix A, in this edition, provides a roadmap that details how readers can follow and use this text.

To fulfill its role as the most respected sports medicine and exercise science professional organization in the world, the American College of Sports Medicine (ACSM) assumed the responsibility of leadership with regard to providing operators of health/fitness facilities with a clearly defined set of recommended practices to promote safe exercise participation. In 1990, in response to guidance given by the ACSM president at that time, Dr. Lyle Micheli, ACSM initiated the process of assembling a team of experts in the academic, medical, and health/fitness fields to develop and write a manual on standards and guidelines for delivering quality physical activity programs and services to consumers. In 1992, the product of the collective efforts of that team was published as a text on standards and guidelines for designing and operating a health/fitness facility. The comprehensive nature of that work was reflected in its 353 separate standards as well as an additional 397 guidelines.

Approximately five years after the first edition of *ACSM's Health/Fitness Facility Standards and Guidelines* was published, a number of steps were undertaken to evaluate the need for and the format of a second edition of the book. The primary action, in this regard, was the appointment of an ad hoc committee of leaders from the medical, exercise science, and health/fitness facility communities to discuss and study the matter. The committee subsequently issued a consensus report that concluded that a second edition of the book was needed to resolve various industry, professional, and consumer-oriented concerns. The committee felt that a second edition of the book would enable the information in the initial text to be updated, while allowing essential features of the publication to be reorganized into what was designed to be a more balanced format. Compared with the first edition, the revised work would place greater emphasis on taking into account the views and input of industry trade organizations and of a wide variety of fitness associations. In this regard, the primary focus was to develop a document that would be more reflective of a true consensus of the health/fitness industry.

In response to the findings of the ad hoc committee, ACSM appointed a committee to develop a second edition of *ACSM's Health/Fitness Facility Standards and Guidelines*, which was published in 1997. In an attempt to gain broader support in the health/fitness industry, the second edition featured a number of major changes from the first edition.

First and foremost, the myriad of standards and guidelines presented in the first edition were consolidated into six standards and approximately 500 guidelines. Responding to a charge given by the ACSM committee that reviewed the first edition, the editorial committee for the second edition reduced the original list of 353 standards that must apply to all health/fitness facilities to six standards. In contrast to the original open-ended tabulation of standards, the six standards identified in the second edition offered a condensed, more realistic focus concerning the standard of care that must be demonstrated by all health/fitness facilities toward their users.

In contrast to the substantial reduction in the number of standards that existed in the second edition, the total number of guidelines increased by more than 20%. Designed to serve as possible tools for health/fitness facility owners and managerial staff to improve their operations, these guidelines set forth design considerations and operating procedures that, if employed, would enhance the quality of service that a facility provides to its users. The guidelines were not intended to be standards of practice or to give rise to duties of care. Finally, the second edition featured an augmented list of appendixes.

In 2004, approximately eight years after the publication of the second edition of *ACSM's Health/Fitness Facility Standards and Guidelines*, a committee of industry-wide representatives and exercise science professionals selected by ACSM recommended that not only would a third edition of this benchmark text be appropriate, but it was also clearly needed. Since research had shown that many health/fitness facilities were not complying with the recommendations set forth in the previous editions of the book, it was determined that it would be helpful if additional clarifications and application-related information were included to accompany each recommendation. Another factor was the need for relevant recommendations concerning the development of the technological advances offered by devices such as automated external defibrillators (AEDs). The third edition of this text was the result of that decision and a by-product of the efforts that followed. In contrast to the first two editions of this book, the third edition was organized into chapters that featured a review and discussion of specific focal points. Each chapter addressed both the standards and guidelines that pertain to a particular issue. All told, the third edition contained nine chapters that addressed specific standards and guidelines in the areas of pre-activity screening; orientation, education, and supervision; risk management and emergency policies; professional

staff and independent contractors; facility design and construction; facility operating practices; facility equipment; and signage. Finally, the number of supplemental materials and forms included in the appendixes was substantially increased over the two previous editions of the book.

Subsequently, ACSM identified a need to produce a fourth edition of this book. Four market forces drove the decision to embark on the compilation and publication of this fourth edition of the standards and guidelines. The first driving force was the Exercise is Medicine initiative, which reflects the growing role of exercise as a medical intervention and the health/fitness club industry's future role as an integral part of the healthcare industry. The evolving role of exercise and fitness in the healthcare arena predicates that health/fitness facilities should establish practices that are appropriate to the needs and interests of the medical and healthcare industry. The second force driving the development of this fourth edition was the involvement of NSF International, the Public Health and Safety Company. In 2007, NSF, an American National Standards Institute (ANSI) accredited standards development organization, embarked on the process of developing a voluntary Health/Fitness Facility Standard (referred to as NSF Standard 341: Health/Fitness Facilities). The to-be-introduced NSF Standard 341 is intended to serve as the foundation for a future voluntary health/fitness facility certification process. A third driving force was the expanding role that government was playing in trying to regulate the practices of the health/fitness facility industry. The role of state governments in areas such as AED legislation and fitness professional licensure and registration for health/fitness facilities was seen as further evidence of the need for the industry to continue expanding its self-regulatory practices. The final driving force for the creation of this fourth edition was related to the evolving nature of the health/fitness industry, particularly the proliferation of new business models and the rapid emergence of former niche business models, such as 24-hour unstaffed facilities, medically integrated facilities, and demographic-specific facilities. These new business models created new demands on the industry for self-regulation.

As with the three previous editions of this text, this book is intended to provide standards and guidelines for pre-activity screening (chapter 1); orientation, education, and supervision (chapter 2); risk management and emergency policies (chapter 3); professional staff and independent contractors (chapter 4); operating practices (chapter 5); facility design and construction (chapter 6); facility equipment (chapter 7); and signage (chapter 8). It is not intended to present general exercise standards and guidelines. The fundamental principles of sound exercise programming and prescription are relatively well documented and readily available elsewhere.

It should be noted that NSF Standard 341: Health/Fitness Facilities, which was still being finalized as this book went to press differs somewhat in both its intended purpose and content from the fourth edition of *ACSM's Health/Fitness Facility Standards and Guidelines*. Specifically, the NSF Standard is a voluntary industry standard that was developed following the protocols used by ANSI accredited standards development organizations, such as NSF, and is intended to serve as the basis for a voluntary health/fitness facility certification for staffed health/fitness facilities. The text, *ACSM's Health/Fitness Facility Standards and Guidelines*, on the other hand, was undertaken in accordance with ACSM's policies and procedures and is intended to provide baseline standards of care, as well as recommended guidelines concerning how all health/fitness facilities, whether staffed *or* unstaffed, can provide a reasonably safe and productive physical activity environment to their members and users. Individuals who are interested in the differences between the NSF Standard for Health/Fitness Facilities and the standards promulgated by ACSM in this edition of its landmark text can refer to appendix L, which provides a comparison of the two sets of standards.

For more information about the NSF Standard, please go to this URL: www.HumanKinetics.com/NSFStandard.

Acknowledgments

The American College of Sports Medicine and the editors of this fourth edition of *ACSM's Health/Fitness Facility Standards and Guidelines* would like to extend their thanks to the members of the editorial board who committed their time and expertise to the writing of this book. Additional thanks are extended to the editors of the three previous editions of this book—Carl Foster, PhD, and Neil Sol, PhD, on the first edition; James A. Peterson, PhD, and Stephen J. Tharrett, MS, on the second edition; and Stephen J. Tharrett, MS, Kyle McInnis, ScD, and James A. Peterson, PhD, on the third edition—for their foresight in helping establish the legacy of this publication.

The editors would also like to extend a special thanks to the ACSM Board of Trustees for their contribution to and involvement in the establishment of this book and its predecessors. For more than 50 years, ACSM has played a leading role in the growth in the level of professionalism exhibited by the industry.

Finally, special thanks are extended to the organizations and professionals that reviewed the draft manuscript for this book and provided the editors with feedback on its content.

Notice and Disclaimer

The primary purpose of the American College of Sports Medicine (ACSM) for developing the previous and current editions of this book is to enhance the safety and effectiveness of physical activity conducted in health/fitness facilities, with the goal of increasing global participation rates in physical activity. To this end, the book will address pre-activity screening practices; orientation, education, and supervision issues; risk management and emergency-procedure practices; staffing issues; operational practices; design issues; equipment issues; and signage issues that have an impact on the safety and effectiveness of physical activity, as engaged in by the general population in health/fitness facilities.

ACSM and its senior co-editors and editorial board, in setting forth standards and guidelines in this book, have done so based on the following definitions for standards and guidelines:

- **Standards.** These are base performance criteria or minimum requirements that ACSM believes each health/fitness facility must meet to provide a relatively safe environment in which physical activities and programs can be conducted. These standards are not intended to give rise to a duty of care or to establish a standard of care; rather, they are performance criteria derived from a consensus of both ACSM leaders and leaders from the health/fitness facility industry. The standards are not intended to be restrictive or to supersede international, national, regional, or local laws and regulations. They are intended to be qualitative in nature. Finally, as base performance criteria, these standards are steps designed to promote quality. They are intended to accommodate reasonable variations, based on local conditions and circumstances.

- **Guidelines.** These are recommendations that ACSM believes health and fitness operators should consider using to improve the quality of the experience they provide to users. Such guidelines are not standards, nor are they applicable in every situation or circumstance; rather, they are tools that ACSM believes should be considered for adoption by health and fitness operators.

ACSM and its senior co-editors and editorial board have designed this book as a resource for those who operate all types of health/fitness facilities, whether they be fully staffed facilities or unstaffed and unsupervised facilities, such as some hotel fitness centers, worksite centers, and commercial 24-hour facilities. Some of the standards and guidelines detailed in this book, in particular those that apply to issues of staffing and supervision or the execution of a practice requiring staffing, may not be applicable to those facilities whose operational model does not include facility staffing.

Despite the development and publication of this book, the responsibility for the design and delivery of services and procedures remains with the facility operator and with others who are providing services. Individual circumstances may necessitate deviation from these standards and guidelines, such as a facility that is not staffed. Facility personnel must exercise professionally derived decisions concerning what is appropriate for individuals or groups under particular circumstances. These standards and guidelines represent ACSM's opinion regarding best practices. Responsibility for service provision is a matter of personal and professional experience.

Any activity, including those undertaken within a health/fitness facility, carries with it some risk of harm, no matter how prudently and carefully services may be provided. Health/fitness facilities are not insurers against all risks of untoward events; rather, their mission should be directed at providing facilities and services in accordance with applicable standards. The standard of care that is owed by facilities is ever changing and emerging. As a consequence, facilities must stay abreast of relevant professional developments in this regard.

By reason of authorship and publication of this document, neither the editors, the contributors, nor the publisher are or are shall be deemed to be engaged in the practice of medicine or any allied health field, the practice of delivering fitness training services, or the practice of law or risk management. Rather, facilities and professionals must engage the services of appropriately trained and/or licensed individuals to obtain those services.

The words *safe* and *safety* are frequently used throughout this publication. Readers should recognize that the use of these terms is relative and that no activity is completely safe.

Definitions

This section of the text provides readers with definitions for the most frequently used words, phrases, and acronyms found throughout the book.

ADA—Refers to the U.S. government's Americans with Disabilities Act, which establishes specific legal requirements for making a building accessible for those with disabilities and physical handicaps.

AED—An acronym for automated external defibrillator, an automated device that can detect the presence and absence of certain cardiac rhythms and deliver a lifesaving electrical shock to the individual.

ASTM International—Originally known as the American Society for Testing and Materials (ASTM), refers to a worldwide voluntary standards development organization for technical standards for materials, products, systems, and services.

barrier protection apparel—Gowns, protective clothing, gloves, masks, and eye shields worn to help protect the staff person from bodily fluids and chemicals.

cardiovascular equipment—Machines that allow an individual to perform whole or partial body movements intended to stimulate the cardiorespiratory system of the individual engaged in using the equipment. Examples include treadmills, elliptical machines, mechanical stair climbers, and indoor cycles.

CPR—An acronym that stands for cardiopulmonary resuscitation, which involves the process of applying chest compressions and, if needed, breaths to assist an individual who is experiencing cardiac arrest.

healthcare professional—Refers to a professional who has education, training, and experience in the provision of healthcare services. In the context of this book, it refers primarily to physicians, registered nurses, nurse practitioners, emergency medical technicians, or others who have received the proper licensing to deliver healthcare services in their respective field of expertise.

health/fitness facility—A facility that offers exercise-based health and fitness programs and services. May include government-based facilities, commercial facilities, corporate-based facilities, hospital-based facilities, and private facilities.

health/fitness facility member—A health/fitness facility user who pays for the regular privilege of engaging in the activities, programs, and services of the facility.

health/fitness facility operator—The owner or management group responsible for the financial and operating activities of a health/fitness facility.

health/fitness facility user—An individual who accesses a facility on one or more than one occasion without purchasing a membership to the facility.

HHQ—An acronym for health history questionnaire, which is a pre-activity screening instrument that is used to collect general health and medical history information about an individual.

HIPPA—An acronym for the U.S. government's Health Information Protection and Portability Act, which provides certain privacy protections to the health information of individuals, including the dissemination of personal health information without the written permission of the individual.

independent contractor—An individual working at a health/fitness facility but not employed by the operator of the facility.

MSDS—An acronym for material safety data sheets. These are sheets that specify data about products and materials per OSHA laws.

OSHA—An acronym for the Occupational Safety and Health Administration of the U.S. government, which oversees the implementation of health and safety regulations required by the government as well as the adherence to these regulations by businesses.

PAD—An acronym for public access defibrillation, a system involving giving the public at large access to AEDs in public and private settings in an effort to bring lifesaving defibrillation to as large a segment of the public as possible.

PAR-Q—An acronym for Physical Activity Readiness Questionnaire, which is a pre-activity screening instrument that helps an individual identify certain health conditions and risk factors that might affect the ability to exercise safely.

personal trainer—An employee or independent contractor of a health/fitness facility whose primary responsibilities are to prescribe exercise for members and users as well as to coach, guide, and supervise members and users while they engage in exercise at a health/fitness facility.

professional staff—Refers to staff who are educated and trained in a professional field, such as fitness or healthcare.

selectorized resistance equipment—Resistance training equipment composed of stacks of weight plates that are attached to a cable and moved over a pulley, allowing users to adjust the amount of weight lifted by selecting the number of plates they desire to lift.

staff—Represents the employees of a health/fitness facility.

staffed health/fitness facility—A health/fitness facility that has employees or independent contractors who work in the facility during all operating hours.

unstaffed health/fitness facility—A health/fitness facility that does not have employees or independent contractors working in the facility during operating hours. This situation can apply for all operating hours or a portion of the facility's operating hours.

variable-resistance equipment—Often the same as selectorized resistance equipment, with the only difference being that instead of a cable run over a standard circular pulley, the pulley is run over a cam-shaped pulley that varies the torque (and hence the level of resistance) of the weight lifted without requiring the actual weight to be changed.

CHAPTER 1

Pre-Activity Screening

The promotion of physical activity is an important focus of both the public health agenda in America and the global health agenda for many nations. In that regard, the time and resources that are devoted to encourage people to be physically active are supported by an ever-accumulating and impressive body of scientific literature that documents the innumerable health benefits of a physically active lifestyle and the potential detrimental effects of sedentary living. As a result of the public health message that individuals should regularly engage in moderate to vigorous physical activity, an increased level of interest and participation in fitness facilities has occurred, including the involvement of adults with diverse health and medical conditions and relatively low levels of cardiorespiratory fitness.

Other factors, such as an aging population in many Western nations, a twin epidemic of obesity and type 2 diabetes in children and young adults around the globe, and efforts to promote physical activity to the "beginner fitness" population, have heightened the need for careful safety policies and procedures that are put into practice at all health/fitness facilities. The primary intent of such policies and procedures is to minimize cardiovascular and/or medical risk for all members and users, including those at greatest potential for cardiovascular risk during exercise due to their age, presence of existing cardiovascular disease, symptoms or risk factors for cardiovascular disease, and any other medical or health concern that might otherwise be exacerbated during exercise participation.

Although most individuals are at a very low risk for an exercise-related cardiovascular event, such as sudden cardiac death or acute myocardial infarction, accumulating scientific evidence suggests the risk of adverse cardiac events is higher during or immediately after vigorous exercise, especially in habitually sedentary individuals who engage in unaccustomed vigorous physical activity (refer to the AHA/ACSM position statement released in 2007, entitled "Exercise and Acute Cardiovascular Events: Placing the Risks Into Perspective" found in appendix J). The risk of a cardiovascular event is highest in persons with a history of cardiovascular disease or individuals who are unaware that they have cardiovascular disease. However, individuals with unrevealed cardiovascular disease are difficult to identify, since many individuals who experience exercise-related cardiovascular emergencies have no previous warning signs.

An important challenge facing health/fitness facility operators is to provide the proper environment for stimulating interest and motivation toward exercise participation, while simultaneously minimizing the potential risk of an adverse medical event occurring during or soon after exercise. A vitally important procedure involved in optimizing safe exercise participation is to identify those individuals who may be at an increased level of risk for such events. The primary step in achieving that objective is to routinely administer a pre-activity health risk assessment on all new members and prospective users. Accordingly, individuals deemed to be at an increased cardiovascular and/or medical risk can be properly evaluated by qualified healthcare providers and steered toward activities that are consistent with their health needs and receive specific recommendations about exercising safely and their potential activity limitations.

Pre-activity screening is the method by which health/fitness facility operators can properly identify those members and users who pose an increased risk of experiencing exercise-related cardiovascular incidents. This procedure is necessary for providing would-be exercisers with appropriate guidelines and recommendations for safe and effective exercise participation. This chapter presents standards (see table 1.1) and guidelines (see table 1.2) pertaining to the use of pre-activity screening tools to help identify those individuals who may be exposed to a greater risk of a cardiovascular event upon engaging in a program of physical activity.

TABLE 1.1   Standards for Pre-Activity Screening

1. Facility operators shall offer a general pre-activity screening tool (e.g., Par-Q) and/or specific pre-activity screening tool (e.g., health risk appraisal [HRA], health history questionnaire [HHQ]) to all new members and prospective users.

2. General pre-activity screening tools (e.g., Par-Q) shall provide an authenticated means for new members, and/or users to identify whether a level of risk exists that indicates that they should seek consultation from a qualified healthcare professional prior to engaging in a program of physical activity.

3. All specific pre-activity screening tools (e.g., HRA, HHQ) shall be reviewed and interpreted by qualified staff (e.g., a qualified health/fitness professional or healthcare professional), and the results of the review and interpretation shall be retained on file by the facility for a period of at least one year from the time the tool was reviewed and interpreted.

4. If a facility operator becomes aware that a member, user, or prospective user has a known cardiovascular, metabolic, or pulmonary disease, or two or more major cardiovascular disease risk factors, or any other self-disclosed medical concern, that individual shall be advised to consult with a qualified healthcare provider before beginning a physical activity program.

5. Facilities shall provide a means for communicating to existing members (e.g., those who have been members for greater than 90 days) the value of completing a general and/or specific pre-activity screening tool on a regular basis (e.g., preferably once annually) during the course of their membership. Such communication can be done through a variety of mechanisms, including but not limited to a statement incorporated into the membership agreement of the facility, a statement on the new-member pre-activity screening form, and a statement on the website.

Pre-activity screening standard 1. Facility operators shall offer a general pre-activity screening tool (e.g., Par-Q) and/or specific pre-activity screening tool (e.g., health risk appraisal [HRA], health history questionnaire [HHQ]) to all new members and prospective users.

The primary purpose of pre-activity screening is to identify those considered to be at risk for an adverse event during exercise and those who would benefit from undergoing an appropriate medical evaluation before starting an exercise program. This objective involves identifying persons with known cardiovascular disease, symptoms of cardiovascular disease, diabetes, other major health concerns, or other risk factors for disease development that may affect safe exercise participation. Screening also identifies persons with known cardiovascular disease or other special medical needs who should ideally participate, at least initially, in a medically supervised program. According to a joint position statement entitled "Exercise and Acute Cardiovascular Events: Placing the Risks into Perspective" by the American Heart Association (AHA) and the American College of Sports Medicine (found in Appendix J), published in *Medicine and Science in Sports and Exercise*, released in 2007, pre-activity screening represents a prudent approach to identifying those individuals who may be at high risk for an acute cardiovascular event during or immediately after vigorous physical activity.

Pre-activity screening tools can be either general (i.e., they provide a generic and simple means of identifying primary cardiovascular disease and/or cardiovascular risk factors) or specific (i.e., they provide a more in-depth approach to identifying preexisting health conditions). The most commonly used general pre-activity screening tool is the Physical Activity Readiness Questionnaire (PAR-Q), which was developed by the Canadian Society for Exercise Physiology. The PAR-Q is a simple one-page questionnaire that asks questions that allow the user, or a facilitator, to easily identify major health conditions, signs, or symptoms suggestive of coronary heart disease, risk factors for cardiovascular disease, medications, or other major medical conditions that may elevate the participant's risk of medical complications during exercise. (Refer to form 1 in appendix C for a sample PAR-Q.)

A commonly used form of a more specific pre-activity screening tool is a health risk appraisal (HRA) questionnaire, of which there are many varieties. HRAs range from simple one-page questionnaires to more complex questionnaires that focus on identifying the health risks associated with an individual's fitness, health, and lifestyle choices. Another commonly used type of a specific pre-activity screening tool is a health history questionnaire (HHQ), of which there are also numerous versions. Because of the greater detail in items that are normally included in HRAs and HHQs, the usefulness of these tools is greatly facilitated when the instruments are utilized with the assistance of fitness or healthcare professionals who have sufficient education and knowledge to interpret the findings and make appropriate recommendations. (Refer to form 2 in appendix C for a sample HHQ.)

Pre-activity screenings (either general or specific) can either be self-administered by the user or conducted by a qualified fitness or healthcare professional. A self-administered general pre-activity screening is most appropriate for health/fitness facilities that are unstaffed during all or part of their operating hours, such as hotel fitness centers, apartment fitness centers, and the ever-growing number of 24-hour unstaffed commercial health and fitness facilities. A self-administered pre-activity screening protocol can range from posting a PAR-Q, with accompanying signage, at the entry to a health and fitness facility to distributing a PAR-Q form to all facility users at their first visit to the facility and having them complete it. Pre-activity screenings, either general or specific, that are facilitated by a fitness or healthcare professional are most suitable for health and fitness facilities that are staffed and focused on providing additional physical activity guidance to users. Furthermore, members and users must be offered the pre-activity screening prior to their participation in the services and programs offered by the facility.

Standards for Pre-Activity Screening

Pre-activity screening standard 2. General pre-activity screening tools (e.g., Par-Q) shall provide an authenticated means for new members, and/or users to identify whether a level of risk exists that indicates that they should seek consultation from a qualified healthcare professional prior to engaging in a program of physical activity.

The objective of this standard is to ensure that if a health/fitness facility operator uses a self-administered pre-activity screening tool for the facility's new members and/or prospective users, that upon completion, the members and users are easily able to determine if their responses indicate they are at a low level of risk, moderate level of risk, or high level of risk for a potential life-threatening event, and that they receive the proper guidance on how to proceed if they desire to reduce the likelihood of a potential life-threatening event based on the results of their self-administered pre-activity screening. Typically, a general pre-activity screening tool will provide the member or user with a quantitative score that can be expressed as low, moderate, or high risk. Furthermore, the pre-activity screening tool will incorporate language that advises the member or user to seek additional professional healthcare advice if the screening results indicate that the person may be at moderate or high level of risk for a potentially life-threatening event upon embarking on a program of physical activity.

Pre-activity screening standard 3. All specific pre-activity screening tools (e.g., HRA, HHQ) shall be reviewed and interpreted by qualified staff (e.g., a qualified health/fitness professional or healthcare professional), and the results of the review and interpretation shall be retained on file by the facility for a period of at least one year from the time the tool was reviewed and interpreted.

Once a member or user has completed a specific pre-activity screening protocol, the facility operator must ensure that the responses are reviewed and interpreted by a qualified member of the facility's staff. A qualified staff person would be a professional who has received fitness professional certification in the health/fitness field, with competency in the area of risk stratification from a third-party accredited organization, such as the National Commission for Certifying Agencies (NCCA), and/or earned a four-year degree from an accredited academic institution in the health/fitness field that provides appropriate training in the area of risk stratification. The American College of Sports Medicine (ACSM) has developed a practical approach to risk stratification that can be used to classify individuals as low, moderate, or high risk. This stratification can be subsequently used to provide recommendations for receiving further evaluation from a qualified healthcare provider. Risk-classification schemes as adapted from ACSM can be used by qualified staff for guiding decisions about making recommendations for medical evaluation are presented in appendix H.

Pre-activity screening standard 4. If a facility operator becomes aware that a member, user, or prospective user has a known cardiovascular, metabolic, or pulmonary disease, or two or more major cardiovascular disease risk factors, or any other self-disclosed medical concern, that individual shall be advised to consult with a qualified healthcare provider before beginning a physical activity program.

It is important for individuals with known cardiovascular disease, metabolic disease, pulmonary disease, or certain identifiable risk factors to receive medical consultation from a qualified healthcare provider before they engage in a moderate to vigorous exercise program. It should be thoroughly explained to these prospective members or users that their disease state and/or existing risk factors could compromise their safety upon engaging in a program of physical activity. In a clear, easy-to-understand manner, the explanation should address why it is in the best interests of such individuals to obtain appropriate healthcare or medical consultation before embarking on their exercise program. The necessity for healthcare or medical consultation is particularly critical for those individuals with predetermined medical conditions (such as coronary heart disease, diabetes, arthritis, and obesity) that involve special needs. In fact, those health and fitness facility operators who primarily (or exclusively) serve such populations should be particularly aware of the value of pre-activity screening involving oversight by qualified personnel.

Pre-activity standard 5. Facilities shall provide a means for communicating to existing members (e.g., those who have been members for greater than 90 days) the value of completing a general and/or specific pre-activity screening tool on a regular basis (e.g., preferably once annually) during the course of their membership. Such communication can be done through a variety of mechanisms, including but not limited to a statement incorporated into the membership agreement of the facility, a statement on the new-member pre-activity screening form, and a statement on the website.

As frequently is the case in the health/fitness facility industry, members will participate in the physical activity programs offered by their particular facility for time periods that can often extend for years. Since the health status of individuals can change during the course of their participation in the activities and services of a health/fitness facility, it is important that members undergo regular pre-activity screenings to ensure that no health condition has arisen since they began exercising that could compromise their health status (e.g., sudden cardiac event, diabetic shock). As a result, it is essential that facility operators communicate to their existing members the importance of receiving a pre-activity screening at least once annually. Facility operators can share this message with their members through a variety of mechanisms, including but not limited to a statement incorporated into the membership agreement of the facility, a statement on the new-member pre-activity screening form, a statement on the website, and posters in the facility.

Standards for Pre-Activity Screening

TABLE 1.2   Guidelines for Pre-Activity Screening

1. Prospective members and/or users who fail to complete the pre-activity screening procedures on request should be permitted to sign a waiver or release that allows them to participate in the program offerings of the facility. In those instances where such members and/or users refuse to sign a release or waiver, they should be excluded from participation to the extent permitted by law.

2. All members or users who have been identified (either through a pre-activity screening or by self-disclosure to a qualified healthcare and/or health/fitness professional on staff) as having cardiovascular, metabolic, or pulmonary disease or symptoms or any other potentially serious medical concern (e.g., orthopedic problems) and who subsequently fail to get consultation should be permitted to sign a waiver or release that allows them to participate in the facility's program offerings. In those situations where such members or users refuse to sign a waiver or release, they should be excluded from participation to the extent permitted by law.

Pre-activity screening guideline 1. Prospective members and/or users who fail to complete the pre-activity screening procedures on request should be permitted to sign a waiver or release that allows them to participate in the program offerings at the facility. In those instances where such members and/or users refuse to sign a release or waiver, they should be excluded from participation to the extent permitted by law.

On occasion, some members or users may not want to participate in the facility's pre-activity screening protocol. While research indicates that completing a pre-activity screening protocol may be beneficial in identifying medical conditions that might expose a member or user to a heightened risk of experiencing a cardiovascular incident during or soon after physical activity, members have the freedom to determine if participating in pre-activity screening is best for them. To reduce the facility's potential liability, it is advisable that such a member or user be asked to sign a waiver or release, where permissible by law, that clearly indicates that the person has been offered a pre-activity screening and that (a) this member or user has been informed of the risks of participation, (b) this member or user has chosen not to follow the guidance provided, (c) this person assumes personal responsibility for his or her actions, and (d) this individual releases the facility from any claims or suits arising from his or her participation. If the member or user signs the waiver or release, that person should be afforded the opportunity to participate in a physical activity program at the facility. If the member or user chooses not to sign the waiver or release, the facility has the option of denying that person the privilege to participate or access to the facility to the extent permitted by law. (Refer to form 6 in appendix C for a sample waiver.)

Pre-activity screening guideline 2. All members or users who have been identified (either through pre-activity screening or by self-disclosure to a qualified healthcare and/or health/fitness professional on staff) as having cardiovascular, metabolic, or pulmonary disease or symptoms or any other potentially serious medical concern (e.g., orthopedic problems) and who subsequently fail to get consultation should be permitted to sign a waiver or release that allows them to participate in the facility's program offerings. In those situations where such members or users refuse to sign a waiver or release, they should be excluded from participation to the extent permitted by law.

When used properly, a pre-activity screening protocol will help determine when a person who may be at increased cardiovascular or medical risk during moderate to vigorous exercise participation could benefit from receiving consultation from a qualified healthcare provider. It is always in the member's or user's and facility operator's best interests to strongly encourage such an individual to obtain the proper medical consultation. It should be noted that instances may occur in which a member or user may not have any known or apparent medical risk factors or symptoms. The facility may still consider it in the best interest of that individual to receive medical consultation before participating in the facility's program offerings.

On occasion, members or users may refuse to obtain recommended medical clearance. When that situation occurs, where legally permissible, the facility should secure a waiver and release that clearly indicates that (a) the users have been informed of the risks of participation and that they have been instructed to obtain medical clearance, (b) they have chosen not to follow the guidance provided, (c) they assume personal responsibility for their actions, and (d) they release the facility operator from any claims or suits arising from their participation. If the member or user signs the waiver or release, that person should be afforded the opportunity to participate in physical activity program offerings at the facility. In the event the member or user chooses not to sign the waiver or release, the facility may choose to deny that individual the privilege of participating in the facility's program offerings or access to the facility to the extent permitted by law.

Guidelines for Pre-Activity Screening

CHAPTER 2

Orientation, Education, and Supervision

The orientation, education, and supervision of members and users in a health/fitness facility are some of the most important obligations a facility operator has to those individuals it serves. Orientation refers to the process of providing each facility member or user with the proper information and guidance to initiate and engage in a program of safe and effective physical activity. Education involves the practice of facility operators providing relevant, up-to-date information to their members and users so that these individuals can make informed decisions about their physical activity and lifestyle practices. Supervision is the process of monitoring the physical activity practices of members and users so that the physical activity environment promotes safe participation.

Several studies have been conducted that indicate that although more than 80% of adults are aware of the benefits of being physically active, a vast majority do not engage in physical activity on a regular basis. Furthermore, research commissioned by the International Health, Racquet and Sportsclub Association (IHRSA) and published in its *2010 Profiles of Success* shows that less than 20% of all Americans are health/fitness facility members, and less than 50% of these individuals use their facility membership at least twice a week. This discrepancy between what Americans know about the benefits of physical activity and their actual behavior patterns, both with regard to exercise in general and participation in the services of health/fitness facilities, serves to reinforce the need for health/fitness facilities to engage in practices that help orient, educate, and supervise users.

This chapter presents standards and guidelines on the orientation, education, and supervision of members and users. Table 2.1 lists the required standards for orientation, education, and supervision; table 2.2 details the recommended guidelines for orientation, education, and supervision.

TABLE 2.1	**Standards for Orientation, Education, and Supervision**

1. Once a new member or prospective user has completed a pre-activity screening process, facility operators shall then offer the new member or prospective user a general orientation to the facility.
2. Facilities shall provide a means by which members and users who are engaged in a physical activity program within the facility can obtain assistance and/or guidance with their physical activity program.

Orientation, education, and supervision standard 1. Once a new member or prospective user has completed a pre-activity screening process, facility operators shall then offer the new member or prospective user a general orientation to the facility.

Once a member has completed a pre-activity screening process, the health/fitness facility operator must then offer the member a general orientation to the facility. A general orientation can take many forms, including any of the following:

- **Group orientation classes.** In facilities that have a low staff-to-user ratio or that have a high volume of member traffic, providing a schedule of orientation classes that members and users can select from can be a viable option. These orientation classes should be offered at various times to allow members and users the opportunity to attend. Among the topics that these orientation classes could cover is basic instruction concerning how members and users should use the various pieces of physical activity equipment that are available in the facility. In addition, these classes could review what resources are available within the facility that can help members and users develop a suitable physical activity program (e.g., personal training services, special fitness classes, fitness media library, online personal training experts). Finally, these classes can also provide an introduction to a general physical activity regimen that members and users can follow.

- **Personal orientation sessions.** The ideal situation for any member is to receive a personal orientation from a qualified fitness professional. This offering allows the individual to receive advice and guidance firsthand from a qualified health/fitness professional. The personal orientation should include general guidelines on physical activity, a personalized exercise regimen that is based on the user's pre-activity screening results and predetermined goals, and a hands-on walk-through of that individual's physical activity regimen.

- **Electronic orientation resources.** A suitable alternative to group orientation classes or personal orientation sessions would be for the facility operator to provide general exercise instruction and facility orientations through electronic media such as the facility's website, in-house computer kiosks, smart phone applications, or similar electronic resources. With the evolution of electronic media and the prevalence of today's members and/or users to access information via the Internet, using this approach to provide general orientations represents a viable alternative. This offering would allow individuals to view specific information on a number of pertinent topics, including how to navigate the facility, tips on properly beginning their exercise program, instruction on the use of the facility's equipment, and a description of the facility's programs and services.

- **Posters and placards.** For the facility operator who may not have the resources to provide personalized orientations or group orientations or the ability to leverage electronic media, the use of posters and placards could serve to provide the type of information and guidance necessary to provide new members and/or users with a general orientation. Posters and placards could provide directions on how to use the facility's equipment, instructions on accessing the facility's services, guidelines on setting up an exercise program, and so on.

> **Orientation, education, and supervision standard 2.** Facilities shall provide a means by which members and users who are engaged in a physical activity program within the facility can obtain assistance and/or guidance with their physical activity program.

While not always possible, the personal instruction and targeted guidance that a qualified health/fitness professional can provide to members will normally result in better safety and productivity than would otherwise be achieved in a given physical activity program. On the other hand, general industry data indicate that only between 5 and 20% of members and users of a facility receive personalized exercise instruction (typically referred to in the industry as *personal training*) on a regular basis. This low level of individualized attention is due, at least in part, to the costs involved in having a health/fitness professional fulfill that particular role. One way that facility operators can help create a greater level of personalized instruction is by offering options that include the following:

- **Complimentary follow-up orientations.** Facility operators can offer new members and current members the opportunity for complimentary 30-minute personal sessions at predetermined intervals (e.g., their 90-day membership anniversary and again at one-year intervals).

- **Fee-based small-group sessions.** Facility operators can offer members the opportunity to purchase at low cost the services of a qualified health/fitness professional who will provide them with initial and ongoing instruction in a semiprivate atmosphere as part of a small group (e.g., two to five members and/or users).

- **Fee-based private sessions.** Facility operators can offer members the opportunity to purchase the services of a qualified health/fitness professional who can provide them with ongoing instruction and guidance.

- **Web-based personalized private instruction.** Facility operators can align themselves (e.g., license, purchase) with one of the Web-based personal training systems that allow members to interact with a qualified fitness professional via e-mail. Many of these programs currently allow a facility's staff to serve as qualified fitness professionals.

TABLE 2.2 Guidelines for Orientation, Education, and Supervision

1. Facilities should provide new and existing members with the opportunity to receive personal instruction and guidance with regard to their physical activity programs.
2. Facilities should provide members with ongoing monitoring of their physical activity programs, including the opportunity to receive guidance on adjusting their physical activity programs.
3. Depending on their targeted audiences, facility operators should consider providing an array of physical activity options to accommodate the physical, emotional, and personal preferences of each user of the facility.
4. Staffed facilities should provide professional health/fitness staff to supervise the fitness floor during peak usage periods.

Orientation, education, and supervision guideline 1. Facilities should provide new and existing members with the opportunity to receive personal instruction and guidance with regard to their physical activity programs.

All factors considered, a qualified health/fitness professional is always a worthwhile option for providing sound advice and individualized feedback on what constitutes an appropriate exercise regimen. Such assistance will typically enhance the effectiveness of the person's physical activity program as well as improve the program's level of safety. Unfortunately, the vast majority of individuals who engage in the services and programs offered by a health/fitness facility do not receive personalized exercise instruction on a regular basis. Among the ways that facility operators can address such a situation is to provide one or more of the following:

• **Complimentary follow-up orientations.** Facilities can offer new members and current members the opportunity for complimentary 30-minute personal sessions at predetermined intervals (e.g., their 90-day membership anniversary and again at one-year intervals).

• **Fee-based small-group sessions.** Facility operators can offer members the opportunity to purchase the services of a qualified health/fitness professional who can provide them with personal instruction and guidance as part of a small group.

• **Fee-based private sessions.** Facilities can offer members the opportunity to purchase the services of a qualified health/fitness professional who can provide them with ongoing instruction and guidance.

• **Web-based personalized private instruction.** Facilities can align themselves (e.g., license, purchase) with one of the Web-based personal training systems that allow members to interact with a qualified fitness professional via e-mail.

Orientation, education, and supervision guideline 2. Facilities should provide members with ongoing monitoring of their physical activity programs, including the opportunity to receive guidance on adjusting their physical activity programs.

Once members and users begin their physical activity programs, their challenge becomes twofold: first, to adhere to the program for a sustained period of time and, second, to achieve their intended program-based health/fitness objectives. Facility operators can assist members with both of these challenges by providing a system of monitoring a person's physical activity. One of the more common physical activity monitoring systems employed by the health and fitness industry involves the use of exercise cards. With exercise cards, members can document their physical activity practices, the results of which can later be reviewed by the facility's professional health/fitness staff. In the event the health/fitness professional sees a need for an adjustment in a member's exercise regimen or notes any unusual circumstances that merit further attention, the member can be contacted and appropriate recommendations can be made.

Another monitoring practice within the health and fitness industry that has gained in popularity in recent years is the use of computer software–based monitoring systems. These systems allow members to record their physical activity efforts in electronic format, either through a computer or mobile handheld device (e.g., cell phone). In the last few years, these software-based monitoring systems have leveraged the accessibility of the Web, allowing individuals to record and track their performance online from anywhere in the world. The results are then reviewed, as needed, by the professional health/fitness staff, who can then follow up with the individual, either electronically or in person. In the event that a facility does not have sufficient staff to implement either of the aforementioned monitoring programs, it could provide its members with either semiannual or annual pre-activity screenings, the results of which could be used to help monitor members on a regular basis.

> **Orientation, education, and supervision guideline 3.** Depending on their targeted audiences, facility operators should consider providing an array of physical activity options to accommodate the physical, emotional, and personal preferences of each user of the facility.

For some individuals, it is not easy to start and stay with a program of physical activity, as evidenced by studies showing more than 50% of new exercisers drop out within 90 days of beginning an exercise program. Research on physical activity attitudes and behavior, as well as market research conducted by the health and fitness industry, clearly shows that one approach does not fit all when it comes to physical activity programs. Specific to their targeted membership (e.g., seniors, women, children, athletes, individuals with special medical conditions), facility operators have a vested interest in getting and keeping their members involved in the activities offered by a particular facility. Accordingly, facility operators need to provide a variety of programs to meet the needs of the marketplace, including the following:

• **Socially-based programs.** Many new and existing members prefer to participate in socially-based physical activity programs. (Note: This type of programming is in the top five preferences for women.) As a result, facilities should consider offering physical activity programs (such as group exercise classes, tennis leagues, group lessons, group personal training, and social events) that feature and foster a component of social interaction in exercise.

• **Competitive-based programs.** Many first-time members and existing members seek a challenge and a competitive outlet within their physical activity pursuits. (Note: This factor is among the top five reasons for men to be motivated to exercise.) As a result, facilities should consider including competitive-based activities, such as sport-related competitions and events (e.g., basketball, racquetball, squash), fitness challenges (e.g., bench press contests, running events), and personal goal-oriented programs (e.g., weight loss) in their offerings.

- **Health and wellness programs.** As stated by members and users, as well as by non-users, among the top reasons for participating is the need for individuals to improve their level of health and well-being. As a result, a facility's offerings should include programs targeted toward health and well-being, such as back education classes, arthritis exercise classes, and nutrition classes. With the advent of the Exercise is Medicine initiative, health and wellness programs will continue to evolve in popularity.

- **Mind–body programs.** Over the past several years, there has been an escalating demand for program offerings that feature a mind–body approach to activity or an approach that focuses on achieving a balance between physical activity, relaxation, and self-awareness. According to market research, women are particularly interested in these types of activities, as are older adults. Among the examples of these types of physical activity programs are Pilates, tai chi, and yoga.

- **Weight loss and weight management programs.** Numerous studies indicate that losing weight is one of the primary reasons many people join health/fitness facilities. This factor, combined with the alarming rise in obesity among Americans and the global community, is more than sufficient reason for facility operators to consider incorporating such popular programs as weight loss, weight management, and nutrition education in their program offerings. Facilities should also consider serving as a resource for their members with regard to the body of knowledge attendant to fitness, health, and wellness. As such, facilities can help keep their members informed about the current facts pertaining to fitness, health, and wellness. Unfortunately, health/fitness facility members, as well as individuals in our society, are constantly bombarded in the media with misinformation about fitness, health, and wellness. As a result, an objective source of information is needed that can help these individuals sort out the information on these topics as it directly applies to their personal needs. Facility operators can provide this information in several ways, including the following:

  - **Communication media.** Facilities can provide their users with important information on fitness and health education through the use of various media. For example, newsletters that have a section devoted to the dissemination of fitness and health information are one viable means of communicating essential information. Websites that have an education page or link to a fitness and health website are another way to help members get the information that they need. The newest trend is to offer members access to social media outlets sponsored by the facility. These social media outlets can range from member and staff blogs on facility websites to special facility pages on one of the many social networking sites (e.g., Facebook, Twitter, YouTube). Finally, a health/fitness facility can use a bulletin board or another similar display on which articles on fitness and health can be posted.

  - **Classes, clinics, and workshops.** Facilities should consider offering classes, clinics, and workshops on specific fitness- and health-related topics to their members and users. For example, a facility could offer a monthly health education seminar series, featuring health and fitness professionals from the community who speak on topics such as cardiovascular health and women's health issues. Another example would be for a facility to have its own professional staff offer a series of workshops on timely and important fitness- and health-related topics, such as weight management, back care education, healthy eating, stress management, and exercise and arthritis.

Orientation, education, and supervision guideline 4. Staffed facilities should provide professional health/fitness staff to supervise the fitness floor during peak usage periods.

During peak periods of usage within a facility (e.g., from 5:00 p.m. to 9:00 p.m.), it is recommended that at least one qualified health/fitness professional be made available on the fitness floor to assist members and users with any questions they may have, to provide guidance when needed, and to respond to any potential emergency situations that might arise. While no precise ratio currently exists for the number of members and users to professional fitness staff, it is suggested that at least one freestanding fitness professional (i.e., an individual who is not engaged in providing users with personalized instruction) should be on the fitness floor for every 100 facility users engaged in exercise in that area on the fitness floor.

CHAPTER 3

Risk Management and Emergency Policies

Risk management refers to the practices and systems that businesses put in place to reduce or limit their exposure to potential liability and financial loss. In the fitness and health club industry, risk management refers to the practices, procedures, and systems by which the club reduces its risk of having an employee, member, or user experience an event that could result in harm (injury or death) to the individual (employee, member, or user) and perhaps later to the business entity itself. Risk management covers practices that range from those that are preventive in nature (such as pre-activity screening and properly caring for equipment) to those practices that are considered a reaction or a recovery-and-response system to untoward events (such as emergency response systems).

This chapter presents standards and guidelines for the risk management and emergency procedures that health/fitness facilities need to consider in order to provide a safe physical activity environment for its employees, members, and users. Some of the standards and guidelines that might otherwise be considered risk management practices, such as pre-activity screening and other operational practices, are addressed in other chapters of this book. Table 3.1 lists the eight required standards for risk management and emergency policies; whereas table 3.3 details the six recommended guidelines for risk management and emergency policies. Table 3.2 contains a listing of the states that have enacted AED legislation.

TABLE 3.1	Standards for Risk Management and Emergency Policies

1. Facility operators must have written emergency response policies and procedures, which shall be reviewed regularly and physically rehearsed at least twice annually. These policies shall enable staff to respond to basic first-aid situations and emergency events in an appropriate and timely manner.

2. Facility operators shall ensure that a safety audit is conducted that routinely inspects all areas of the facility to reduce or eliminate unsafe hazards that may cause injury to employees and health/fitness facility members or health/fitness facility users.

3. Facility operators shall have a written system for sharing information with members and users, employees, and independent contractors regarding the handling of potentially hazardous materials, including the handling of bodily fluids by the facility staff in accordance with the guidelines of the U.S. Occupational Safety and Health Administration (OSHA).

4. In addition to complying with all applicable federal, state, and local requirements relating to automated external defibrillators (AEDs), all facilities (i.e., staffed or unstaffed) shall have as part of their written emergency response policies and procedures a public access defibrillation (PAD) program in accordance with generally accepted practice, as highlighted in this section.

5. AEDs in a facility shall be located within a 1.5-minute walk to any place an AED could be potentially needed.

6. A skills review, practice sessions, and a practice drill with the AED shall be conducted a minimum of every six months, covering a variety of potential emergency situations (e.g., water, presence of a pacemaker, medications, children).

7. A staffed facility shall assign at least one staff member to be on duty during all facility operating hours who is currently trained and certified in the delivery of cardiopulmonary resuscitation and in the administration of an AED.

8. Unstaffed facilities must comply with all applicable federal, state, and local requirements relating to AEDS. Unstaffed facilities shall have as part of their written emergency response policies and procedures a PAD program as a means by which either members and users or an external emergency responder can respond from time of collapse to defibrillation in four minutes or less.

Risk management and emergency policies standard 1. Facility operators must have written emergency response policies and procedures, which shall be reviewed regularly and physically rehearsed at least twice annually. These policies shall enable staff to respond to basic first-aid situations and emergency events in an appropriate and timely manner.

Having an emergency response system is critical to providing a safe environment for members, users, and staff, as well as being a sound practice in risk management. For health/fitness facilities, emergency response systems must be developed in order to provide the highest reasonable level of safety for members and users. Emergency policies, procedures, and practices for health/fitness facilities, as presented and discussed in this chapter, are derived from recommendations published jointly in 1998 and 2002 by ACSM and AHA. (Refer to appendixes H and I.)

Many of these recommendations are identified and discussed in this chapter in the context of standards for health/fitness facilities in 2011 and beyond. However, it is acknowledged that the types of health/fitness facilities vary markedly, from facilities that are unsupervised to medically supervised clinical exercise centers. Such facilities often serve different aims and clientele, may or may not have organized program offerings, and may or may not have qualified staff. Thus, beyond the standards offered in this chapter, facilities needing assistance in matters of preparing emergency policies, procedures, and practices relevant to their setting will find the contents of the 1998 and 2002 ACSM/ AHA publications to be helpful resources. Among the more crucial elements attendant to incorporating emergency response systems in a facility are the following:

- Facility operators should use local healthcare or medical personnel to help them develop their emergency response program. Most local emergency medical services (EMS) will assist a facility in developing its response program. Facilities can also pay for the services of a physician, registered nurse, or certified emergency medical technician to guide the development of their emergency response program.

- The emergency response system must address the major emergency situations that might occur. Among those situations that might arise are those medical emergencies that are reasonably foreseeable with the onset of moderate or more intense exercise, such as hypoglycemia, sudden cardiac arrest, heart attack, stroke, and heat illness, and those injuries that are orthopedic in nature. The response system must also address other foreseeable emergencies not necessarily associated with physical activity, such as fires, chemical accidents, and natural disasters.

- The emergency response system must provide explicit steps or instructions on how each emergency situation will be handled and the roles that should be played by first, second, and third responders to an emergency. In addition, the emergency response system needs to provide locations for all emergency equipment (e.g., telephone for 911 or other contact information for EMS, the location for all emergency exits, and the most favorable access ways for EMS personnel) as well as the steps necessary for contacting the local EMS.

- The emergency response system must be fully documented (i.e., staff training, emergency instructions), and pertinent information must be kept in an area that can be easily accessed by the club staff. In addition, the emergency response system needs to be reviewed with facility staff on a regular basis.

- The emergency response system must be physically rehearsed at least two times per year, with notations maintained in a log that indicate when the rehearsals were performed and who participated.

- The emergency response system must address the availability of first-aid kits and other medical equipment within the facility.

- The emergency response system should identify a local coordinator (e.g., a staff person who is responsible for a facility's overall level of emergency readiness).

Risk management and emergency policies standard 2. Facility operators shall ensure that a safety audit is conducted that routinely inspects all areas of the facility to reduce or eliminate unsafe hazards that may cause injury to employees and health/ fitness facility members or health/fitness facility users.

It is critical that facility operators remain aware of conditions within their facility that could pose an increased risk to their employees, members, and users. To this end, it is critical that facility operators develop an audit and/or inspection process that allows them to regularly check the safety of their facility. This audit process can be as simple as a checklist of the critical safety practices that must be in place, which allows the staff to verify that all the proper safety practices are being followed. The goal is for the operator to establish a schedule for inspecting the facility to determine adherence to the specific safety practices that the facility has put in place to protect the employees, members, and users. In all cases, the result of each inspection or audit should be maintained on file by the facility operator for a period of at least three years.

Risk management and emergency policies standard 3. Facility operators shall have a written system for sharing information with members and users, employees, and independent contractors regarding the handling of potentially hazardous materials, including the handling of bodily fluids by the facility staff in accordance with the guidelines of the U.S. Occupational Safety and Health Administration (OSHA).

The health and fitness industry often encounters situations that can expose members and users, employees, and independent contractors to materials that OSHA considers dangerous. Employees and independent contractors, such as custodial staff, lifeguards, locker room and health/fitness staff, and others, may be exposed to chemicals and materials that are potentially hazardous, such as cleaning agents, paints, and lubricants. Those individuals who are in enclosed areas where air circulation is limited can be exposed to particle matter, such as debris resulting from sanding, drilling, or similar activity. To comply with OSHA guidelines and reduce the risk to members and users and to staff, facilities need to consider the following actions:

- Make sure that the material safety data sheet (MSDS) for every chemical and agent used in the facility is posted in a location for all workers to view (e.g., intranet site, posters).

- Provide an MSDS binder (e.g., hard copy or electronic) for each staff person to review, and have each person sign appropriately to signify that he or she has reviewed the information and understands the issues.

- Store all chemicals and agents in proper locations. Ensure that these materials are stored off the floor and in an area that is off limits to users. These areas should also have locks to prevent accidental or inappropriate entry.

- Provide regular training to staff in the handling of these items.

- Post the appropriate signage to warn members and users that they may be exposed to these hazardous agents.

The health and fitness facility industry often is faced with circumstances that may expose its users and staff to various bodily fluids. Almost every human interaction associated with this industry has the potential to result in contact with bodily fluids. As such, the possibility exists that disease-producing organisms may be present in those fluids. Consequently, exposure carries a risk of infection. The OSHA standard on blood-borne pathogens addresses how such fluids must be handled to minimize risks of infection. Many facility operators fail to realize that even the handling of towels presents an increased risk of exposure to bodily fluids such as blood or perspiration. Some key steps that every facility can take to minimize risk in this area include the following:

- Provide appropriate training for staff. Make sure that all staff are taught how to handle bodily fluids. OSHA provides training materials, as do other organizations.

- Provide literature to staff on the handling of bodily fluids.

- Make sure that the staff members who are handling towels, cleaning or picking up papers, and cleaning exercise equipment wear surgical-style latex gloves (note that for those individuals who are allergic to latex, gloves made of nonallergic material should be provided). Staff that has to handle bar soap or razors also need to be provided with latex gloves or a similar type of gloves.

- Make sure that the facility has a system for disposing of items containing bodily fluids. If the facility has razors, then a biohazard container for disposing of them must be provided. If facility personnel are washing towels, bleach must be used, since it will kill most pathogens carried in bodily fluids.

If blood is visible, it must be cleaned off immediately with bleach or a similar agent while staff wear barrier protection apparel (e.g., impermeable gloves). All cleaning materials and all fluids must be disposed of in biohazard containers. Untrained staff should not be permitted to handle these materials or fluids. Full details on the OSHA Hazard Communication Standard are included in appendix B, supplement 5.

Risk management and emergency policy standard 4. In addition to complying with all applicable federal, state, and local requirements relating to automated external defibrillators (AEDs), all facilities (i.e., staffed and unstaffed) shall have as part of their written emergency response policies and procedures a public access defibrillation (PAD) program in accordance with generally accepted practice, as highlighted in this section.

A PAD program uses AEDs, which are sophisticated computerized machines that are simple to operate and enable a layperson with minimal training to administer this potentially lifesaving intervention. AEDs allow a layperson responding to an emergency to use the AED device, which can detect certain life-threatening cardiac arrhythmias and then administer an electrical shock that can restore the normal sinus rhythm. AEDs are the third step in the American Heart Association's (AHA's) renowned Chain of Survival concept, after alerting EMS and administering CPR. Helpful suggestions concerning the important features of PAD programs and resources to assist facilities with integrating the PAD program in their emergency response protocols may be found at the AHA website at www.americanheart.org.

Research reviewed by the AHA shows that the delivery speed of defibrillation, as offered by an AED, is the major determinant of success in resuscitative attempts for ventricular fibrillation (VF) cardiac arrest (the most common type of cardiac arrest). Survival rates after VF decrease 7% to 10% with every minute of delay in initiating defibrillation. A survival rate as high as 90% has been reported when defibrillation is administered within the first minute of cardiac arrest, but survival decreases to 50% at 5 minutes, 30% at 7 minutes, 10% at 9 to 11 minutes, and 2% to 5% after 12 minutes.

Communities that have incorporated AED use in their emergency practices have shown significant improvements in survival rates for individuals who have experienced cardiac events. For example, in the state of Washington, the survival rate increased from 7% to 26%; in Iowa, the survival rate increased from 3% to 19%. Some public programs have reported survival rates as high as 49% when an AED is used promptly. The American Heart Association is a strong proponent of having AEDs as accessible to the public as possible. The use and application of AEDs in a public setting are detailed in the American Heart Association's 2010 *Guidelines for CPR and ECC*.

Some key elements of an effective PAD program are as follows:

- Every site with an AED should strive to get the response time from collapse caused by cardiac arrest to defibrillation to four minutes or less.

- The Food and Drug Administration (FDA) requires that a physician prescribe an AED before it can be purchased. The AHA strongly recommends that a physician, licensed to practice medicine in the community in which the health/fitness facility is located, should provide the oversight of the facility's emergency response system and AEDs. In most cases, the company from which an AED is purchased will assist the facility with identifying a physician to provide these services. Physician oversight refers to the following:
  - Prescribing the AED
  - Reviewing and signing off on the emergency plan
  - Witnessing at least one rehearsal of the emergency plan and indicating so in writing
  - Providing standing orders for use of the AED
  - Reviewing documentation from any instances when the emergency plan is initiated and the AED is used

- A club's emergency plan and AED plan should be coordinated with the local EMS provider. (Note: Most of the product providers offer this assistance.) Coordinating with the local EMS provider refers to the following:
  - Informing the local EMS provider that the club has an AED or AEDs
  - Informing the local EMS provider of the location of each AED at the facility
  - Working with the local EMS provider to provide ongoing training of the facility's staff in the use of the AED
  - Working with the local EMS provider to provide monitoring and review of AED events

- All incidences involving the administration of an AED must be recorded and then reported to the physician who is providing AED oversight as soon as possible, but no longer than one day. (The Health Information Protection and Portability Act [HIPPA] does not allow medically sensitive information to be released to anyone other than the medical director.)

- Each club should have an AED program coordinator who is responsible for all aspects of the emergency plan and the use of the AED, as outlined in the standards of care detailed in this book.

- All staff likely to be put in a situation where they may have to administer an AED should be appropriately trained and certified in a course that incorporates the administration of the AED from an accredited training organization. Currently, the AHA and the American Red Cross (ARC) provide AED basic life support training and certification that involve a minimum of four hours of direct-contact training. AHA training and certification lasts approximately two years, while the corresponding ARC program lasts for about one year. Records of training and retraining should be maintained in staff personnel records or as part of the documentation of the facility's emergency response system.

An effective and rapid PAD system actually depends on bystanders participating in rapid recognition of potential sudden cardiac arrest and the deployment of an AED for possible use. For this reason, health/fitness facilities are encouraged to work with their medical directors and EMS support systems to carefully define prudent and appropriate ways to include all facility members and users in the emergency response system. This process may include consideration of how members and users might be involved, directly or indirectly, in accessing and deploying an AED and at what point during the emergency protocol that step may be required (e.g., sudden collapse of an individual and no staff member is immediately present). Written instructions might be provided to every member or user concerning the approved PAD program in the facility, what the bystander or user response should be in an emergency, and where the AED is located. Likewise, orientation of new facility members might include a simple printed information card indicating the location of pertinent emergency response postings in the facility; the locations of the emergency telephone and AED; which staff members may need to be employed to handle an emergency; and where their offices are located, should EMS activation be needed.

The orientation for new users could also include visits to locations in the facility to point out areas that are listed on the emergency response information card they have been given. While it is recognized that developing an appropriate way to involve all users in a PAD program will need careful and thoughtful consideration, this process may help to reduce the time between cardiac arrest and defibrillation, when the cause of collapse is ventricular fibrillation, especially in medium to large facilities during those times when member, user, and staff presence is minimal.

The AED should be monitored and maintained according to the manufacturer's specifications on a daily, weekly, and monthly basis, and all information in that regard should be carefully documented and maintained as part of the facility's emergency response system records. AEDs provide this function through an automated process.

At the present time, the use of AEDs in the health and fitness industry has remained somewhat controversial. In 2003, for example, the International Health, Racquet and Sportsclub Association (IHRSA) released a position statement on AEDs that indicated that while the Association thought that health/fitness facilities should consider the installation of an AED, it did not think that AEDs should be mandated for them. The AHA and ACSM released a joint position statement in 2002 that recommended the implementation of AEDs in health/fitness facilities (appendix I). As of December 2010, only 11 states (Arkansas, California, Illinois, Indiana, Louisiana, Massachusetts, Michigan, New Jersey, New York, Oregon, and Rhode Island) have passed legislation that requires health/fitness facilities to have AEDs. Table 3.2 provides a summary of the various states with AED legislation and some of the general aspects of that legislation. It should be noted that in

TABLE 3.2 States With AED Legislation for Health/Fitness Facilities*

State	Protection from civil liability	Require employee CPR/AED training	Size requirement for facility	Financial assistance provided to facilities	Law covers unstaffed facilities
Arkansas	✓	✓			✓
California	✓	✓			
Illinois	✓	✓	✓		
Indiana	✓	✓			✓
Louisiana	✓	✓			
Massachusetts	✓	✓			✓
Michigan	✓	✓		✓	
New Jersey		✓		✓	
New York	✓	✓	✓		
Oregon	✓		✓		
Rhode Island	✓	✓			✓

* As of December 2010.

four states, legislation allows unstaffed facilities (e.g., 24-hour key-card access facilities, hotel-based facilities) to use AEDs without having trained employees present. As of December 2010, the state of Wisconsin had legislation pending regarding AEDs in the health/fitness setting, and it should be expected that in the future, additional states will pass legislation requiring health/fitness facilities to provide access to AEDs. In reality, most of the premier health/fitness facility operators in the United States have already made AEDs an integral part of their emergency response systems. It should be noted that AED use in health/fitness facilities is not yet a global issue, as the European Union has yet to establish legislation in this regard.

Risk management and emergency policy standard 5. AEDs in a facility shall be located within a 1.5-minute walk to any place an AED could be potentially needed.

The American Heart Association, in its *Guidelines for Emergency Cardiac Care*, indicates that while a facility should be able to get a response time from collapse caused by cardiac arrest to defibrillation of four minutes or less, the best means of achieving this objective is to provide AEDs in locations that staff or the public can reach within a 1.5-minute walk. If an individual were to walk at a rate of 3 mph (4.8 km/h), this effort would involve a distance of slightly over 500 ft (150 m). As a result, a facility operator should consider the time needed to reach various sites within its facilities from various locations and then identify those locations that would allow its staff, members, or the public to access an AED within a 1.5-minute time span. If a facility occupies multiple floors, it might be wise to consider locating an AED on each floor to ensure that the device can be reached within the appropriate time limitation.

Risk management and emergency policy standard 6. A skills review, practice sessions, and a practice drill with the AED shall be conducted a minimum of every six months, covering a variety of potential emergency situations (e.g., water, presence of a pacemaker, medications, children).

A skills review and practice sessions with the AED should be held every six months, as recommended by the AHA's Emergency Cardiac Care Committee and a number of international experts. While some experts recommend practice drills as often as once a quarter, no research exists that would indicate less frequent rehearsal poses any greater risk to the members and users of a health/fitness facility. The key takeaway of this standard for health/fitness facility operators is that conducting a physical rehearsal (e.g., practice drills) at least every six months will help ensure that the staff of the facility are prepared to respond to cardiac events that take place on the premises of the facility.

Risk management and emergency policy standard 7. A staffed facility shall assign at least one staff member to be on duty during all facility operating hours who is currently trained and certified in the delivery of cardiopulmonary resuscitation and in the administration of an AED.

AEDs must be applied by an individual who has received the proper training and certification in the delivery of cardiopulmonary resuscitation and the administration of an AED. Since the administration of an AED requires the presence of a trained and certified individual, it only makes sense that staffed facilities have at least one staff person who is qualified to administer the AED.

Over the past several years, a proliferation has occurred of unstaffed health/fitness facilities that provide members and users with 24/7 access to facilities without the presence of staff. In these situations, since the facility operator will be unable to provide trained and certified staff, the facility must therefore provide a means for either members and users or external healthcare responders who are properly trained and certified to respond and administer an AED. It should be noted that of the 11 states requiring AEDs in health/fitness settings, only 4 have laws that cover unstaffed facilities (see table 3.2).

Risk management and emergency policy standard 8. Unstaffed facilities must comply with all applicable federal, state, and local requirements relating to AEDs. Unstaffed facilities shall have as part of their written emergency response policies and procedures a PAD program as a means by which either members and users or an external emergency responder can respond from time of collapse to defibrillation in four minutes or less.

Since unstaffed facilities will not have staff present who could witness an event, they must provide a means by which other members and users who witness an event can activate the emergency response system and/or respond independently with regard to administering an AED to a member or user who has succumbed to an actual or perceived cardiac event. To this end, unstaffed facilities need to provide a means of monitoring members and users in the facility, and then when an event occurs, provide a means by which the member or user can be attended to within a four-minute time period from the time of collapse. Examples of approaches an unstaffed facility could take in this regard include the following:

- Provide video monitoring of the facility (e.g., install a system that enables staff to monitor video of all appropriate areas of the facility during all unstaffed hours) so that any incident can be observed immediately.

- Provide "panic buttons" in various locations throughout the facility so that a member or user, including the individual who may be experiencing an event, can notify emergency responders by pushing the button.

- Provide telephone or other communication devices in various locations throughout the club so that a member or user, including the individual who may be experiencing an event, can notify emergency responders.

- Have AEDs in the facility placed in visible locations, along with simple directions on how to access and administer the AED in the event a member or user witnesses a cardiac event or collapse.

> **TABLE 3.3   Guidelines for Risk Management and Emergency Policies**
>
> **1.** Facilities should use waivers of liability and/or assumption of risk documents with all facility members and users.
>
> **2.** A facility that delivers or prescribes physical activity programs, primarily or exclusively, to members and users who are considered at an elevated risk for experiencing a health-related event because of their participation in physical activity (e.g., users over the age of 50, individuals with coronary risk factors, diabetes, or clinical obesity) should have a medical director, a medical liaison, or a medical advisory committee provide assistance in reviewing the facility's physical activity screening and programming protocols as well as its emergency response protocols.
>
> **3.** Facilities should provide the appropriate level of supervision and monitoring for each of the physical activity areas in the facility.
>
> **4.** All physical activity areas should have a clock, a chart of target heart rates, and a chart depicting ratings of perceived exertion to enable members and users to monitor their level of physical exertion.
>
> **5.** A facility should extend to each employee on staff the opportunity to receive training and certification in first aid and the use of CPR and an AED.
>
> **6.** Facilities should have an incident report system that provides written documentation of all incidents that occur within the facility or within the facility's scope of responsibility. Such reports should be completed in a timely fashion and maintained on file, according to the regulatory statute of limitations for the location in which the facility does business.

Risk management and emergency policies guideline 1. Facilities should use waivers of liability and/or assumption of risk documents with all facility members and users.

An expressed assumption of risk is a legal document that the members and users sign, which indicates that they are aware of the risks associated with their participation in the various physical activity programs offered by the facility and that they are knowingly accepting full responsibility for their decision to participate in those activities and are releasing the facility from any and all responsibility for their participation. A waiver is a legal document that, by voluntarily signing, members and users give up, or waive, their right to institute a claim or litigation. These documents, when properly drafted and executed, are enforceable in many states. The waivers, however appropriate and legal, do not necessarily bar a user from filing a claim against a facility or from the possibility of litigation if the plaintiff's attorney advises the client that a viable cause of action exists. Thus, facilities must practice due diligence in the safe delivery of services in accordance with applicable standards and guidelines. An assumption of risk or waiver should be prepared by an attorney and should address the following factors at a minimum:

- The facility's programs and services to which the member or user has access and might use to pursue a program of physical activity

- The risks involved in participating in any moderate or more intense exercise, including the risk of a cardiac event or even death

- A statement that the member or user is aware of the risks involved, that the facility has explained those risks thoroughly, and that the user is willing to accept those risks

- The member's or user's willingness to accept all responsibility for participation in light of the information he or she has been provided and that the member or user is accepting complete responsibility for his or her actions and is releasing the facility from any and all liability associated with the decision, including the facility's ordinary negligence

The use of a waiver should be regular practice for all facilities. Ideally, all members and users should complete and sign a waiver form upon joining a facility. Previous editions of *ACSM's Health/Fitness Facility Standards and Guidelines* and the 1998 IHRSA Health and Safety Standards indicate that the use of waivers should be a standard practice for health/fitness facility operators.

The health and fitness industry has numerous positions that require specific personal licensing, registration, or certification for employment. In these instances, applicants must possess the required credentials to be considered qualified to serve in a particular position-specific capacity. Facilities can limit their risk in this situation by ensuring (both at the time of employment or contract signing and during the course of work) that each employee's and independent contractor's credentials are valid and current. If an individual serving in a position that requires special education, training, registration, or licensure is found not to have the appropriate credentials, then the facility is exposing itself to considerable risk. Examples of positions where credentials need to be checked at the time of employment or contract signing and on an ongoing basis thereafter include fitness instructor, fitness director, personal trainer, group exercise instructor, massage therapist, esthetician, and dietitian. Chapter 4 provides details on some of the specific education, certification, licensing, and experience requirements for several of the professional roles that exist within a facility and the expectations for documenting current qualifications of employees.

Risk management and emergency policies guideline 2. A facility that delivers or prescribes physical activity programs, primarily or exclusively, to members and users who are considered at an elevated risk for experiencing a health-related event because of their participation in physical activity (e.g., users over the age of 50, individuals with coronary risk factors, diabetes, or clinical obesity) should have a medical director, a medical liaison, or a medical advisory committee provide assistance in reviewing the facility's physical activity screening and programming protocols as well as its emergency response protocols.

With the emergence of Exercise is Medicine (an initiative undertaken by ACSM), it makes sense for health/fitness facility operators to consider creating a medical advisory committee or retaining, either on a voluntary or fee basis, a medical liaison or medical director. The rationale for this guideline is that by having either a medical advisory committee, medical liaison, or medical director, facility operators can receive guidance and advice that can enhance the overall safety of their operation as well as help position their organizations as part of the healthcare continuum. It should be noted that the Medical Fitness Association, in its *Standards and Guidelines for Medical Fitness Center Facilities* (found in appendix K), has a standard that actually mandates the presence of a medical director and/or medical advisory committee.

Creating a medical advisory committee can be as simple as putting together a group of medical and healthcare professionals from the community who volunteer their time to review the facility's policies and practices pertaining to pre-activity screening, member and user fitness assessment, member and user exercise program prescription, and emergency response protocols. A medical advisory committee might meet as frequently as quarterly or as infrequently as annually. If a health/fitness facility operator considers the creation of a medical advisory committee, the advisory panel should work closely with both the local medical and the legal community in order to help protect both the medical advisory committee members and appropriate facility personnel.

Having a medical liaison or medical director, while definitely not a necessity, is a good practice for facilities that are involved in the medical fitness arena. Having a medical liaison could involve retaining a physician or other qualified healthcare professional (e.g., licensed registered nurse, licensed nurse practitioner) on a consulting basis to provide general guidance and direction on how to structure the programs and services to safely service populations who are experiencing certain medical or health conditions that are traditionally the responsibility of healthcare professionals.

Risk management and emergency policies guideline 3. Facilities should provide the appropriate level of supervision and monitoring for each of the physical activity areas in the facility.

An appropriate level of supervision and monitoring is highly dependent upon the types of activities offered by a health/fitness facility as well as by the members and users it serves. If a facility serves a population of members and users who are older and are experiencing a variety of health problems, this situation would require more supervision and monitoring than a facility that serves a young, apparently healthy population. Likewise, if a facility has a basketball court, a fitness center, a pool, and a group exercise studio, each of these areas has different needs with regard to the level of supervision and monitoring. For example, a basketball court may not require supervision except when an organized league is being conducted, while a pool area may require two lifeguards to be on duty at all times. It is the responsibility of facility operators to know the nature of their facility and the type of audience they serve and then provide the appropriate level of supervision and monitoring, based on their business model.

Risk management and emergency policies guideline 4. All physical activity areas should have a clock, a chart of target heart rates, and a chart depicting ratings of perceived exertion to enable members and users to monitor their level of physical exertion.

The monitoring of heart rate during physical exertion is one of the most accurate and meaningful ways of monitoring members' and users' level of exertion while they're engaged in physical activity. In those cases in which heart rate monitoring does not effectively monitor the level of physical exertion (e.g., individuals on certain medications, those with certain cardiovascular conditions), the use of perceived exertion provides an accurate and easily understood means of monitoring an individual's level of physical exertion. Heart rate monitoring and monitoring of perceived exertion are important elements of providing members and users with a safe and effective physical activity environment. To this end, it is recommended that facility operators provide members and users with the appropriate devices so that they can monitor their heart rate (e.g., clocks, timers) and their level of perceived exertion (e.g., perceived exertion chart, perceived exertion scale) as well as compare them to the appropriate measures of heart rate and perceived exertion for individuals of a similar age and gender (e.g., perceived exertion charts, heart rate charts).

Risk management and emergency policies guideline 5. A facility should extend to each employee on staff the opportunity to receive training and certification in first aid and the use of CPR and an AED.

While the relevant standard requires staffed health/fitness facilities to have only one AED trained and certified staff member on duty during operating hours, those operators who wish to provide a higher level of safety for their members and users should consider providing all staff with training and certification in the use of an AED. This level of commitment from a health/facility operator would help ensure that at least one trained and certified staff person is available at all times who can appropriately respond to a cardiac emergency in the facility.

Risk management and emergency policies guideline 6. Facilities should have an incident report system that provides written documentation of all incidents that occur within the facility or within the facility's scope of responsibility. Such reports should be completed in a timely fashion and maintained on file, according to the regulatory statute of limitations for the location in which the facility does business.

Facilities that desire to reduce their potential liability and provide their staff, members, and users with a safer work and physical activity environment should make the use of a written incident report system a part of their daily operating practice. An incident report system provides a means for the facility to document all incidents that involve individuals within the facility (e.g., staff, members and users, and independent contractors).

A properly completed written document of an incident, whether it is a minor slip and fall or a major medical emergency, allows the facility to obtain information that can assist in the response to the incident and serves as a resource for any future requests for information about the incident. The information collected in an incident report becomes privileged information that can be released only to the proper authorities, after approval of the involved parties. A proper incident report system should incorporate a written report that is completed by a qualified and responsible employee of the facility. Ideally, this report should be completed as soon as possible after an incident has occurred. The incident report system might include the following:

- A written incident report form (see forms 20 and 30 in appendix C for sample forms). At a minimum, the completed form should contain the following types of information:
  - Day, date, and time of the incident
  - Location of the incident
  - Person(s) involved in the incident
  - Witnesses to the incident
  - Staff responding to the incident
  - Actions taken when responding to the incident
  - Outcomes of the incident

- A team review of the incident should be conducted by qualified staff. The day after an incident occurs, it is advisable for the involved responders to review the report and resulting actions with facility management to assess the facility's response and to determine if further actions need to be taken.

- In the event of a major incident, the incident report should be forwarded to the facility's insurance carrier.

- It is always advisable for management to follow up with the involved parties to address any outstanding issues and make sure that the situation has been handled appropriately.

CHAPTER 4

Professional Staff and Independent Contractors for Health/Fitness Facilities

The fitness and health club industry is a people-intensive industry. As such, several recent surveys, including Profiles of Success, published annually by the International Health, Racquet and Sportsclub Association (IHRSA), indicate that many health/fitness facilities allocate upward of 40% of their gross revenues to wages, salaries, and benefits. Not surprisingly, when a business allocates 40% or more of its resources to one specific factor, that area takes on critical importance to the success of that organization. The health and fitness industry is no different. Employees and independent contractors help to create and sustain the experiences that individuals undergo as a result of their membership in a particular health/fitness facility. Consequently, the employees and independent contractors in the industry have both a direct and an indirect effect on a health/fitness facility's level of operating success. Among the most critical of these employee and independent-contractor groups are the fitness and healthcare professionals who provide guidance, personal and group instruction, and supervision for facility users.

The most important role that staff and independent contractors who serve in the industry as fitness and healthcare professionals have is to ensure that a health/fitness facility's members' and users' experiences involving that facility are positive, including everything that should be done and could reasonably be done to ensure that members and users are exposed to the enumerable benefits of being physically active. Furthermore, these professionals also have responsibility for providing a physical activity environment within a health/fitness facility that is reasonably safe. This responsibility includes the ability to respond to potential health-related emergencies.

Accordingly, fitness and healthcare professionals must have the necessary competencies for fulfilling their various roles and responsibilities. These competencies normally involve some combination of education, training, certification, and hands-on experience. Among fitness and healthcare professionals who are most likely to interact with facility members and users on a regular basis, help oversee essential program offerings, and assume supervisory responsibility for key initiatives within the facility are the fitness directors, fitness instructors, personal trainers, group exercise instructors, physical activity instructors, and lifestyle counselors. In addition to the aforementioned group of fitness and healthcare professionals, other key employees and independent contractors are the medical and healthcare liaisons, such as physical therapists, chiropractors, and physicians, who may interact directly or indirectly with the health/fitness facility members and users during the course of the physical activity programs being conducted.

This chapter presents standards and guidelines regarding the competency expectations for the aforementioned core group of professional staff and independent contractors. Table 4.1 provides a list of the three required standards for professional staff and independent contractors; tables 4.2 and 4.3 offer an overview of the combination of training (education, certification, and experience) that would constitute the reasonable expectation that a person would be competent to fulfill the professional demands of a particular position. Table 4.4 provides a list of the major professional certifications that are available in the health and fitness industry. Table 4.5 provides a general summary of states that have or are considering legislation with regard to the registration or licensure of personal trainers, and table 4.6 provides a list of guidelines for professional staff and independent contractors for health/fitness facilities. Table 4.7 provides a general summary of certifications available for health/fitness professionals serving special populations.

TABLE 4.1 Standards for Health/Fitness Facility Professional Staff and Independent Contractors

1. The health/fitness professionals who have supervisory responsibility and oversight responsibility for the physical activity programs and the staff who administer them shall have an appropriate level of professional education, work experience, and/or certification. Examples of health/fitness professionals who serve in a supervisory role include the fitness director, group exercise director, aquatics director, and program director.

2. The health/fitness and healthcare professionals who serve in counseling, instruction, and physical activity supervision roles for the facility shall have an appropriate level of professional education, work experience, and/or certification. The primary professional staff and independent contractors who serve in these roles are fitness instructors, group exercise instructors, lifestyle counselors, and personal trainers.

3. Health/fitness and healthcare professionals engaged in pre-activity screening or prescribing, instructing, monitoring, or supervising of physical activity programs for facility members and users shall have current automated external defibrillation and cardiopulmonary resuscitation (AED and CPR) certification from an organization qualified to provide such certification. A certification should include a practical examination.

Professional staff and independent contractors standard 1. The health/fitness professionals who have supervisory responsibility and oversight responsibility for the physical activity programs and the staff who administer them shall have an appropriate level of professional education, work experience, and/or certification. Examples of health/fitness professionals who serve in a supervisory role include the fitness director, group exercise director, aquatics director, and program director.

The fitness and healthcare professionals who have supervisory and oversight responsibility for the physical activity programs and related services and the staff who administer them shall have an appropriate level of professional education, work experience, and/or certification.

The primary fitness and healthcare professionals who serve in a supervisory role are the fitness director, group exercise director, aquatics director, and program director. Table 4.2 provides examples of what might be considered an appropriate blend of professional education, certification, and work experience for some of the primary supervisory positions within the health and fitness industry.

TABLE 4.2	Recommended Competency Criteria for Program Supervisors in the Health and Fitness Industry		
Professional position	Professional education	Professional certification	Professional experience
Aquatics director	4-year degree in fitness, exercise science, or a related field from an accredited college* or university is recommended but not required.	Certification in advanced lifesaving and water safety from a nationally recognized organization is recommended. Certification as a pool operator from either a national (NSPI) or local organization or government agency is recommended.	Minimum of 3 years' experience as a lifeguard, water safety instructor, or swim instructor is recommended.
Fitness director	4-year degree in fitness or a health-related field from an accredited college* or university is recommended.	Fitness instructor, personal trainer, or health/fitness specialist certification from a nationally recognized and accredited* certifying organization is recommended.	Minimum of 3 years' experience as a fitness professional working in the fitness and health industry in a health/fitness facility is recommended.
Group exercise director	2 years post–high school education in fitness, health, recreation, or a related field from an accredited college* or university is recommended but not required.	Group exercise instructor certification from a nationally recognized and accredited* certifying organization is recommended.	Minimum of 3 years' experience as a group exercise instructor working in the fitness and health industry in a health/fitness facility is recommended.
Program director	4-year degree in fitness, exercise science, or a related field is recommended.	Certification in fitness, group exercise, or a related recreational field from a nationally recognized and accredited* certifying organization is recommended.	Minimum of 3 years' experience working as an instructor or supervisor of physical activity or recreation programs is recommended.

*The term *accredited* refers to certification programs that have received third-party approval of their certification procedures and practices from an appropriate agency, such as the National Commission for Certifying Agencies (NCCA), or from institutes of higher education whose curriculum has received accreditation from the Commission on Accreditation of Allied Health Education Programs (CAAHEP).

Professional staff and independent contractors standard 2. The health/fitness and healthcare professionals who serve in counseling, instruction, and physical activity supervision roles for the facility shall have an appropriate level of professional education, work experience, and/or certification. The primary professional staff and independent contractors who serve in these roles are fitness instructors, group exercise instructors, lifestyle counselors, and personal trainers.

Table 4.3 details examples of what might be considered the appropriate blend of professional education, certification, and work experience for some of the relevant positions in the health and fitness industry. Table 4.4 offers an overview of some of the major certifications available to these professionals in the health and fitness industry.

TABLE 4.3	Recommended Competency Criteria for Instructors, Counselors, and Personal Trainers in the Health and Fitness Industry		
Professional position	**Professional education**	**Professional certification**	**Professional experience**
Fitness instructor	4-year degree in fitness, exercise science, or a related field is recommended, with 2 years of college education in the field as a recommended minimum.	Fitness instructor or personal trainer certification from a nationally recognized and accredited* certifying organization is recommended.	Minimum of 6 months' experience working as a fitness instructor or personal trainer is preferred.
Group exercise instructor	High school education is required, and 2 years of college education in fitness, exercise science, dance, or a related field is recommended but not required.	Group exercise instructor or leader certification from a nationally recognized and accredited* certifying organization is recommended.	Minimum of 100 hours' experience observing and teaching group exercise or fitness classes is preferred.
Lifestyle counselor	4-year degree in fitness, health, or a related field is recommended.	Fitness instructor or personal trainer certification from a nationally recognized and accredited certifying agency is required. Additional certification from such organizations in lifestyle management, behavior change, or a similar area is recommended.	Minimum of 1 year's experience working as a fitness instructor or personal trainer, with at least 100 hours' experience in lifestyle counseling, is recommended but not required.
Personal trainer	4-year degree in fitness, exercise science, or a related field is recommended, with 2 years of college education in the field as a recommended minimum.	Fitness instructor or personal trainer certification from a nationally recognized and accredited* certifying organization is recommended.	Minimum of 6 months' experience, working as a fitness instructor or personal trainer is preferred.

*The term *accredited* refers to certification programs that have received third-party approval of their certification procedures and practices from an appropriate agency, such as the National Commission for Certifying Agencies (NCCA), or from institutes of higher education whose curriculum has received accreditation from the Commission on Accreditation of Allied Health Education Programs (CAAHEP).

With regard to what would be considered an appropriate level of certification for personal trainers, IHRSA in 2006 adopted a position statement that IHRSA clubs should retain only personal trainers who have received certification from an organization whose certification had received third-party approval of its certification procedures. In the last few years, several U.S. state legislatures have initiated legislative efforts to regulate the qualifications necessary to become a personal trainer. As of December 2010, eight U.S. states have initiated legislative action toward the registration (i.e., requiring a certain level of education and certification) or licensure of personal trainers (see table 4.5), with one state, California, having passed legislation through its Senate, with final Assembly approval pending. A ninth state, Kansas, is also considering legislation in this arena. This legislative movement toward requiring either licensure or registration of personal trainers continues to collect momentum, thereby increasing the need for the health/fitness industry to establish greater conformity in the regulation of personal trainer qualifications. In Europe, the European Health and Fitness Association (EHFA) has proposed a set of competency standards for two levels of fitness professionals. The first competency level applies to instructors who provide general guidance and instruction either in a group setting (e.g., group exercise instructors) or within the gym or fitness center (e.g., fitness instructors), and the second level applies to personal trainers who provide more personalized instruction for the members and users of European health/fitness facilities.

TABLE 4.4   Major Certifications Available in the Health and Fitness Industry

Organization	Sample certifications available
American College of Sports Medicine	Personal trainer, health/fitness specialist
American Council on Exercise	Group fitness instructor, personal trainer, lifestyle and weight management consultant
Aerobics and Fitness Association of America	Primary group exercise, personal fitness trainer
National Academy of Sports Medicine	Certified personal trainer, performance enhancement specialist
National Strength and Conditioning Association	Certified personal trainer, certified strength and conditioning specialist

TABLE 4.5   States With Pending or Inactive Legislation Pertaining to Personal Trainer Registration and/or Licensure*

State	Focus of legislation
California	Personal trainer registration. Senate Bill 1043 based on NCCA accredited certifications. Passed Senate and now in the Assembly.
District of Columbia (DC)	Personal trainer licensing. Bill pending.
Georgia	Personal trainer licensing. Senate Bill 441 introduced in February 2010.
Louisiana	Licensing of exercise physiologists already in place, and personal trainer licensure being considered.
Massachusetts	Personal trainer licensing. Senate Bill 870 in committee.
Maryland	Personal trainer licensing. House Bill 747 introduced in 2010.
New Jersey	Personal trainer licensing. Senate bill 695.
New Hampshire	Personal trainer licensing. House Bill 1313 introduced in 2010.

* As of December 2010.

Professional staff and independent contractor standard 3. Health/fitness and healthcare professionals engaged in pre-activity screening or prescribing, instructing, monitoring, or supervising of physical activity programs for facility members and users shall have current automated external defibrillation and cardiopulmonary resuscitation (AED and CPR) certification from an organization qualified to provide such certification. A certification should include a practical examination.

The majority of fitness and healthcare professionals working in a fitness facility environment will never need to respond to a life-threatening cardiovascular event, but the ability to respond in a competent manner is at the core of providing members and users with a reasonably safe physical activity environment. Since those health/fitness professionals engaged in pre-activity screening, exercise prescription, exercise instruction, and exercise activity monitoring are more likely to be in the presence of members and users who are engaged in moderate to vigorous physical activity, it is imperative that they have training and certification in CPR and AED administration from a recognized certifying organization such as the American Heart Association or American Red Cross. In its 2010 publication, *Guidelines for CPR and ECC*, the American Heart Association clearly indicates that those responding to a sudden cardiac event must be certified in AED and CPR.

TABLE 4.6	Guidelines for Health/Fitness Facility Professional Staff and Independent Contractors

1. Facility operators should consider having health/fitness professionals who have the appropriate level of professional education and/or certification to assess and prescribe physical activity for individuals with special needs.
2. Facility operators should consider having all staff members trained and certified in cardiopulmonary resuscitation and AED administration.
3. Facility operators should perform criminal background checks on employees and independent contractors who have responsibilities that involve working with youth or whose responsibilities involve personal contact with members and users or other employees in an unsupervised environment.

Professional staff and independent contractor guideline 1. Facility operators should consider having health/fitness professionals who have the appropriate level of professional education and/or certification to assess and prescribe physical activity for individuals with special needs.

Over the past 5 to 10 years, an ever-increasing number of individuals considered as having a health condition that limits their ability to safely participate in physical activity programs are engaging in services offered by health/fitness facilities. It is not uncommon to find members and users with physical disabilities (such as blindness or loss of mobility in one or more limbs) and/or medical conditions (such as diabetes, COPD, heart disease, cancer, cerebral palsy, muscular dystrophy) participating in exercise programs under the supervision of health/fitness professionals in the health/fitness facility environment. In these instances, it is prudent for health/fitness facility operators to consider having the health/fitness professional demonstrate the proper level of professional competency, as evidenced by the appropriate professional education and/or certification. Table 4.7 provides examples of several industry certifications for health/fitness professionals who are working with different special populations.

TABLE 4.7	Professional Certifications Available for Health/Fitness Professionals Serving Special Populations	
Organization	**Sample certification**	**Special population**
American Council on Exercise	Advanced fitness specialist	Preventive rehabilitation and postrehabilitation for individuals at risk of or recovering from metabolic, cardiovascular, or pulmonary disease
American College of Sports Medicine	ACSM/NCPAD (National Center on Physical Activity and Disability) certified inclusive trainer	Individuals with physical, sensory, or cognitive disability
	ACSM/ACS certified cancer exercise trainer	Individuals with cancer or recovering from cancer
	Registered clinical exercise physiologist	Individuals under the care of a physician and rehabilitating from cardiovascular, pulmonary, metabolic, neuromuscular, neoplastic, immunologic, hematologic, musculoskeletal, and other diseases
	Clinical exercise specialist	Individuals under the care of a physician and rehabilitating from cardiovascular, pulmonary, or metabolic diseases
National Academy of Sports Medicine	Corrective exercise specialist	Injury prevention and recovery
Arthritis Foundation	Arthritis foundation exercise program leader and trainer certification	Individuals with arthritis

Professional staff and independent contractor guideline 2. Facility operators should consider having all staff members trained and certified in cardiopulmonary resuscitation and AED administration.

In the health and fitness industry, most fitness and healthcare professionals, as a rule, have AED and CPR certification. On occasion, however, some professionals do not. Accordingly, a health/fitness facility should always take steps to ensure that at least one person is on duty at all times when the facility is open who has the training and certification to administer first aid, CPR, and/or AED. Because the first responders to many of the emergencies that occur in a health/fitness facility may not be fitness professionals but instead are frontline, non–fitness professional staff, facilities should consider providing every employee with the opportunity to be properly trained in first aid, AED, and CPR. It is in everyone's best interests for a health/fitness facility to give its employees the opportunity to be properly trained in these essential emergency practices. The more health/fitness facility staff who receive AED and CPR training and certification, the greater the likelihood that facility operators will be able to respond to emergencies in a timely manner.

Professional staff and independent contractor guideline 3. Facility operators should perform criminal background checks on employees and independent contractors who have responsibilities that involve working with youth or whose responsibilities involve personal contact with members and users or other employees in an unsupervised environment.

Any employee or independent contractor whose responsibilities include working one on one with a member or user in an unsupervised environment should be subject to a criminal background check. Members and users put their trust in a facility, particularly its staff and representatives. As such, it is an obligation to make sure that its employees and contractors are not individuals whose past history suggests that they are a threat to the safety and security of the members and users. Background checks allow an operator to identify if anything in an employee's or contractor's past history (e.g., criminal activity of any kind) would present a threat to the safety of the members and users. Criminal background checks can be conducted through local law enforcement authorities (in this instance, they tend to provide evidence of local criminal activity only) or through regional and national companies (these organizations often provide information on a national scope) that offer such services to private and public institutions. In the case of employees and/or independent contractors who work with youth, it is suggested that background checks also look into any possible criminal record related to offenses against children.

CHAPTER 5

Health/Fitness Facility Operating Practices

Operating practices refer to those administrative policies, practices, procedures, and systems that a facility uses to deliver its products and services to members and users in a manner that is consistent with the vision and business model of the facility. Operating practices can range from the policies governing scheduling appointments to the practice of conducting orientations for new members. The more formalized these operating practices are, the more likely the facility will consistently deliver its products and services in the desired manner.

In the health and fitness industry, a number of excellent operating practices exist. As a result, no one best method for operating a health/fitness facility can be determined. Instead, there are benchmarks or best practices that clearly define the parameters of what health/fitness facility operators need to do in order to run their business successfully. The most successful facility operators tend to divide operations into two important components: operating standards and systems. Operating standards are the basic expectations that a facility has for delivering a specified practice. They serve as a framework for staff concerning the facility's mission statement. The systems are the tools that staff can use to meet the operational standards or expectations.

This chapter presents the standards and guidelines for a health/fitness facility's operating practices. Table 5.1 lists eight standards for health/fitness facility operations. This chapter is not intended as an in-depth look at facility operations. In contrast, it is designed to provide a template regarding operational practices that health/fitness facilities can use as appropriate. Table 5.2 highlights information on temperature, humidity and appropriate precautions for saunas, steam rooms and whirlpools. Table 5.3 highlights appropriate chemistry levels for pools per the recommendations of the National Spa and Pool Institute (NSPI). Table 5.4 lists the four recommended guidelines pertaining to operating practices of health/fitness facilities. Tables 5.5 and 5.6 highlight general cleaning and disinfecting guidelines for various facility areas.

| TABLE 5.1 | Standards for Health/Fitness Facility Operating Practices |

1. Facilities shall have an operational system in place that monitors, either manually or technologically, the presence and identity of all individuals (e.g., members and users) who enter into and participate in the activities, programs, and services of the facility.

2. Facilities that offer a sauna, steam room, or whirlpool shall have a technical monitoring system in place to ensure that these areas are maintained at the proper temperature and humidity level and that the appropriate warning systems and signage are in place to notify members and users of any risks related to the use of these areas, including subsequent unsafe changes in temperature and humidity.

3. Facilities that offer members and users access to a pool or whirlpool shall provide evidence that they comply with all water-chemistry safety requirements mandated by state and local codes and regulations.

4. A facility that offers youth services or programs shall provide evidence that it complies with all applicable state and local laws and regulations pertaining to their supervision.

5. When a child is under direct staff supervision of a facility, as a participant in either an organized activity or in an ongoing facility program, or is just under temporary staff supervision while the parent or legal guardian is using the facility, the responsible staff person shall have ready access to the child's basic medical information, which has been previously collected from the parent as part of the child registration process.

6. The registration policy of a facility that provides child care shall require that parents or guardians of all children left in the facility's care complete a waiver, an authorization for emergency medical care, and a release for the children whom they leave under the temporary care of the facility.

7. The facility shall require that parents and guardians provide the facility with names of persons who are authorized by the parent or legal guardian to pick up each child. The facility shall not release children to any unauthorized person, and furthermore, the facility shall maintain records of the date and time each child checked out and was dropped off and the name of the person to whom the child was released.

8. Facilities shall have written policies regarding children's issues, such as requirements for staff providing supervision of children, age limits for children, restroom practices, food, and parental presence on site. Facilities shall inform parents and guardians of these policies and require that parents and guardians sign a form that acknowledges that they have received the policies, understand the policies, and will abide by the policies.

Health/fitness facility operating practices standard 1. Facilities shall have an operational system in place that monitors, either manually or technologically, the presence and identity of all individuals (e.g., members and users) who enter into and participate in the activities, programs, and services of the facility.

The ability to identify all individuals entering the facility and the members and users who are participating in the various physical activity programs offered by the facility is important for at least three reasons. First, by knowing who enters the facility, the staff members at the facility can enhance the level of safety in the facility by ensuring that only those individuals with privileges have access to the facility. Second, by having knowledge of which members and users are in the facility, the staff at the facility can respond more effectively to potential emergency situations. Third, having knowledge of who is using the facility at any given time can influence the development of both staffing and supervision schedules for each area of the facility, which in turn can provide a safer physical activity environment for the members and users.

Monitoring systems can be either manual or electronic. Manual systems involve having members and users sign in whenever they enter the facility. With a manual system, most facilities expect the members and users not only to sign in but also to record the time of their entry. Electronic (e.g., computer software based) systems require that the members and users either present an identification card to the facility or use some other form of personal identification (e.g., fingerprint, eye scan) to record their visits. The computerized systems automatically record the time of a person's entry and maintain records of every visit.

Health/fitness facility operating practices standard 2. Facilities that offer a sauna, steam room, or whirlpool shall have a technical monitoring system in place to ensure that these areas are maintained at the proper temperature and humidity level and that the appropriate warning systems and signage are in place to notify members and users of any risks related to the use of these areas, including subsequent unsafe changes in temperature and humidity.

Saunas, steam rooms, and whirlpools are all potentially high-risk areas to members and users because of the high temperatures and humidity that are generated in these spaces. A facility's failure to maintain these three areas at what are considered safe temperature and humidity levels can further expose members and users to harmful conditions, such as hyperthermia, heat exhaustion, heatstroke, and cardiovascular emergencies. Even when maintained at the proper temperature, these three areas can still result in dangerous consequences if individuals are not warned of the associated risks and precautions that go with their use. While events such as heart attack and stroke are very rare, events such as orthostatic syncope (i.e., a condition where a person feels dizzy or faint from the venous pooling of blood that occurs upon changing from a supine to upright position) or heat exhaustion and heatstroke have a higher likelihood of occurring. Table 5.2 provides an overview of the recommended temperature ranges and precautions for saunas, steam rooms, and whirlpool areas.

TABLE 5.2   Recommended Temperatures and Precautions for Saunas, Steam Rooms, and Whirlpools

Facility zone	Recommended temperature range	Typical cautionary wording
Sauna	160-170 °F (71-77 °C)	• Limit use to no more than 10 minutes at one time. • Wait at least 10 minutes after completing exercise before entering. • If you are pregnant, have heart disease, have kidney disease, are on certain medications for cardiovascular disease, and/or have other medical issues that could be adversely affected by high heat, do not use. • Exposure to high temperatures for an extended period of time can result in heat exhaustion, heatstroke, heart attack, and, on occasion, death.
Steam room	100-110 °F (38-43 °C)	• Limit use to 10 minutes at one time. • Wait at least 10 minutes after completing exercise before entering. • If you are pregnant, have heart disease, have kidney disease, are on certain medications for cardiovascular disease, and/or have other medical issues that might be adversely affected by high heat, do not use. • Exposure to high temperatures for an extended period of time can result in heat exhaustion, heatstroke, heart attack, and, on occasion, death.
Whirlpool	102-105 °F (39-41 °C)	• Limit use to 10 minutes at one time. • Wait at least 10 minutes after exercise before entering. • If you are pregnant, have heart disease, have kidney disease, are on certain medications for cardiovascular disease, and/or have other medical issues that might be adversely affected by high heat, do not use. • Exposure to high temperatures for an extended period of time can result in heat exhaustion, heatstroke, heart attack, and, on occasion, death.

Health/fitness facility operating practices standard 3. Facilities that offer members and users access to a pool or whirlpool shall provide evidence that they comply with all water-chemistry safety requirements mandated by state and local codes and regulations.

In most states, either the state or local municipality with governing authority establishes standards for the proper water chemistry. Most state and local codes provide minimums for the various chemical levels of the water. Facility operators can also refer to the National Spa and Pool Institute (NSPI) for more thorough information on the proper water chemistry for pools and whirlpools (spas). Table 5.3 provides an overview of the ranges recommended by the NSPI for the most critical water chemical levels in a pool.

TABLE 5.3 Recommended NSPI Guidelines for Pool Chemistry

Water chemical	Min	Ideal	Max
Free chlorine	1.0	1.0 to 3.0	3.0
Combined chlorine (ppm)	None	None	0.2
Bromine (ppm)	2.0	2.0-4.0	4.0
Ph	7.2	7.4-7.6	7.8
Total alkalinity (ppm)	60	80-100	180
Calcium hardness (ppm)	150	200-400	500-1,000+
Cyanuric acid (ppm)	10	30-50	150

* ppm refer to parts per million

Health/fitness facility operating practices standard 4. A facility that offers youth services or programs shall provide evidence that it complies with all applicable state and local laws and regulations pertaining to their supervision.

In all states, laws exist governing the supervision of children left under the care of a business. In certain states, facilities, including health/fitness facilities, must be licensed by the state in order to supervise a child in the absence of a parent or guardian. In many states, if the parent is on the premises and the period the child is left under the temporary supervision of the facility operator is less than a few hours (*note:* because of the variance in laws, codes, and regulations that exist between localities, readers are advised to check into the statutes that are applicable to their geographic area), then licensure is not required. Properly caring for and supervising any children who are present in a health/fitness facility are critical responsibilities. Accordingly, facilities that offer some form of children's programs or services must make sure they are in compliance with all federal and state laws and regulations.

Health/fitness facility operating practices standard 5. When a child is under direct staff supervision of a facility, as a participant in either an organized activity or in an ongoing facility program, or is just under temporary staff supervision while the parent or legal guardian is using the facility, the responsible staff person shall have ready access to the child's basic medical information, which has been previously collected from the parent as part of the child registration process.

When a child is in the exclusive control of a facility's staff (i.e., the parent or guardian is not in the facility), or when the child is under temporary supervision of the facility's staff (i.e., in a child care area while the parent is participating in activities of the facility), basic medical information must be obtained by the facility and available to the person or persons in the facility who are responsible for the child. This step requires that the facility staff work with the parents to collect relevant information, which should focus on any allergies, illnesses, and any other special medical conditions that the child may have. This medical information should be kept on file for a period of at least one year and updated on an annual basis if the child continues to be left under the exclusive or temporary supervision of the facility's staff.

Health/fitness facility operating practices standard 6. The registration policy of a facility that provides child care shall require that parents or guardians of all children left in the facility's care complete a waiver, an authorization for emergency medical care, and a release for the children whom they leave under the temporary care of the facility.

Each parent or guardian must complete a waiver and release for the children whom they leave in the facility's care. In some states, parents and guardians cannot disclaim, waive, or release their responsibility for their children's rights; therefore, facility operators should check the relevant laws in their state. In addition to a waiver, facility operators need to have the parents or guardians complete an authorization of medical care and release for the children whom they are leaving under the exclusive or temporary care of the facility operator. The authorization of medical care allows the facility operator in a medical emergency, especially when the parent or guardian cannot be reached, to undertake the appropriate medical emergency response to ensure the child's safety and well-being.

Health/fitness facility operating practices standard 7. The facility shall require that parents and guardians provide the facility with names of persons who are authorized by the parent or legal guardian to pick up each child. The facility shall not release children to any unauthorized person, and furthermore, the facility shall maintain records of the date and time each child checked out and was dropped off and the name of the person to whom the child was released.

A facility must have an appropriate system for ensuring that children are dropped off and picked up by authorized individuals. Authorized individuals are those people whom the parents and/or guardians have indicated in writing are allowed to drop off their child or pick up their child from under the exclusive or temporary care of the facility's staff. An appropriate record of the drop-off and pickup of the child should be maintained at all times.

Health/fitness facility operating practices standard 8. Facilities shall have written policies regarding children's issues, such as requirements for staff providing supervision of children, age limits for children, restroom practices, food, and parental presence on site. Facilities shall inform parents and guardians of these policies and require that parents and guardians sign a form that acknowledges that they have received the policies, understand the policies, and will abide by the policies.

Facilities need to have written policies regarding potentially critical children's issues, such as age limits, restroom practices, food, and parental presence on site. Parents must be informed of these policies and, subsequently, must sign a form indicating that they have received these polices, understand the policies, and will abide by the policies. All staff and independent contractors who work in situations where they may be alone with children must undergo both a criminal background check and a child-abuse clearance, where available.

TABLE 5.4   Guidelines for Health/Fitness Facility Operating Practices

1. Facilities that are staffed during all operating hours should have a manager on duty (MOD) or supervisor on duty (SOD) schedule that specifies which professional staff person has supervisory responsibility overseeing all operating activities during the hours that the facility is open.
2. Facility operators who operate under a staffed business model should provide the proper level of qualified staffing in nonactivity areas to assist in serving the members and users and providing support to emergency response situations that might arise.
3. Facilities that are unstaffed during some or all operating hours, and therefore have periods in which no supervision is offered, should provide the appropriate signage to communicate to members and users that the facility is unsupervised, the inherent risks in using the facility, and what steps the members and users should take in the event of a witnessed emergency situation.
4. Facilities should have a written system for cleaning and disinfecting the various areas in the facility.

Health/fitness facility operating practices guideline 1. Facilities that are staffed during all operating hours should have a manager on duty (MOD) or supervisor on duty (SOD) schedule that specifies which professional staff person has supervisory responsibility overseeing all operating activities during the hours that the facility is open.

In the health and fitness industry, extensive operating hours often are the norm; many staffed facilities are open for members and users 24 hours a day. With such extensive operating hours, it is important that facilities provide a professional staff person to serve as a manager or supervisor on duty (e.g., MOD) during all operating hours. During that person's designated shift, the MOD serves as the point person for member, user, and staff issues and, more importantly, as the lead person in any emergency response situations that might arise. The MOD needs to be trained and certified in AED, CPR, and first aid as well as thoroughly versed in the facility's basic operating procedures.

Health/fitness facility operating practices guideline 2. Facility operators who operate under a staffed business model should provide the proper level of qualified staffing in nonactivity areas to assist in serving the members and users and providing support to emergency response situations that might arise.

As discussed in chapter 3, some facilities operate with minimal or no staffing, while others function in a fully staffed manner. If the facility operator has chosen a staffed business model, then, in addition to the professional fitness staff whose primary responsibilities vary from person to person, depending on the assigned role within the facility, facility operators should also ensure proper staffing levels for nonphysical activity settings, including the front desk, child care areas, housecleaning, locker rooms, and administrative offices.

Health/fitness facility operating practices guideline 3. Facilities that are unstaffed during some or all operating hours, and therefore have periods in which no supervision is offered, should provide the appropriate signage to communicate to members and users that the facility is unsupervised, the inherent risks in using the facility, and what steps the members and users should take in the event of a witnessed emergency situation.

Over the past several years, the number of health/fitness facilities that operate under an unstaffed business model (e.g., some hotel fitness centers, some corporate fitness centers, many 24-hour key-card access commercial fitness centers) has increased, especially in the United States. If a health/fitness facility operator chooses to operate a business model that is unstaffed, then the facility operator should make every effort to provide the appropriate signage that clearly indicates to members and users that they are assuming personal responsibility for engaging in the use of the facility without staff supervision, and that as a result, certain risks (pertaining to the unsupervised environment) exist with which they should be prepared to deal.

Health/fitness facility operating practices guideline 4. Facilities should have a written system for cleaning and disinfecting the various areas in the facility.

According to research sponsored by IHRSA, consumers see facility cleanliness as one of the top five factors that influence their decision to join a particular facility. From a safety perspective, the failure to maintain a proper schedule of cleaning and disinfecting facility areas and equipment can lead to the spread of germs that can cause illness. Accordingly, a facility should develop and adhere to a written schedule for cleaning (and disinfecting, where applicable) all areas and relevant equipment in the facility. Furthermore, a facility should maintain written records in that regard. Tables 5.5 and 5.6 provide samples of recommended cleaning and disinfecting procedures for various areas of a health/fitness facility.

TABLE 5.5 Sampling of Recommended Cleaning and Disinfecting Procedures for Fitness and Group Exercise Zones

Facility area	Cleaning activity	Frequency
Fitness floor (gym)	• Remove trash.	• Daily
	• Dust all horizontal surfaces.	• Daily
	• Clean and disinfect vinyl pads on equipment.	• Daily
	• Clean and disinfect equipment frames.	• Daily
	• Vacuum carpets and clean stains.	• Daily
	• Spot-clean mirrors.	• Daily
	• Wash and disinfect hard floor surfaces, including all rubber floor surfaces.	• Daily
	• Clean heating, ventilation, and air conditioning (HVAC) vents.	• Monthly
	• Clean light fixtures.	• Monthly
	• Vacuum and clean under all equipment.	• Monthly
	• Fully clean mirrors and glass surfaces.	• Monthly
	• Clean carpets.	• Quarterly or annually
	• Clean wall surfaces thoroughly.	• Annually
Group exercise studio	• Remove any trash.	• Daily
	• Dry-mop wood floors.	• Daily
	• Dust all horizontal surfaces.	• Daily
	• Spot-clean mirrors and glass surfaces.	• Daily
	• Clean mirrors thoroughly.	• Daily
	• Wet-mop wood floors.	• Daily
	• Clean HVAC ducts.	• Monthly
	• Clean light fixtures.	• Monthly
	• Clean audio equipment.	• Monthly
	• Wash solid walls.	• Monthly
	• Refinish wood floor surfaces.	• Annually

TABLE 5.6 Sampling of Recommended Cleaning and Disinfecting Procedures for Gymnasiums and Sports Courts

Facility area	Cleaning activity	Frequency
Gymnasium or sports court	• Remove trash.	• Daily
	• Dry-mop and dust floors.	• Daily
	• Dust all horizontal surfaces.	• Daily
	• Spot-clean all glass surfaces.	• Daily
	• Clean all glass surfaces thoroughly.	• Weekly
	• Tack or wet-mop the wood floors.	• Weekly
	• Clean HVAC filters.	• Monthly
	• Clean light fixtures.	• Monthly
	• Refinish wood floors.	• Every 2 years as needed

CHAPTER 6

Health/Fitness Facility Design and Construction

According to research sponsored by the International Health, Racquet and Sportsclub Association (IHRSA), consumers weigh a facility's equipment and space offerings as one of the primary factors affecting their decision to join a club. According to IHRSA studies, facilities can be separated into two basic types: fitness-only facilities and multipurpose facilities. While these two broad categories provide a basis for identifying the two primary types of health/fitness facilities, each of these two categories can be further separated into subcategories, based on the type of business operation within a particular facility.

Fitness-only facilities are defined as facilities that offer space specifically for the pursuit of fitness activities. Typically, these facilities consist of activity areas for cardiovascular equipment, variable-resistance circuit equipment, free weight equipment, and, in some instances, studios for group exercise. These facilities also include several common spaces, such as locker rooms and reception areas.

The major subcategories of fitness-only facilities are exercise studios, free weight gyms, apartment fitness rooms, corporate fitness centers, and express facilities (e.g., Anytime Fitness, Snap Fitness, Curves for Women, McFit). Exercise studios typically have one or two group exercise studios, a reception area, and locker rooms. Free weight gyms, on the other hand, normally provide a large free weight area, a reception area, and locker rooms. Fitness centers in apartment buildings and hotels generally are located in a somewhat limited space and typically feature a few pieces of cardiovascular and variable-resistance equipment. Corporate fitness centers range from small areas that contain a few pieces of variable-resistance equipment and cardiovascular equipment to larger spaces that hold complete lines of cardiovascular, variable-resistance, and free weight equipment. In fact, many of the smallest fitness-only facilities often occupy less than 1,000 sq ft (94 sq m) of space.

Multipurpose facilities are defined as facilities that offer both fitness facilities and one or more recreational spaces such as racquet courts, pools, gymnasiums, spas, and outdoor recreational areas. The majority of multipurpose facilities range in size from 40,000 to 100,000 sq ft (12,192 to 30,480 sq m).

The various subcategories of multipurpose health/fitness facilities include those with racquet courts only, pools only, gymnasiums only, facilities with tennis courts, and facilities with a blend of several activity areas. As a rule, almost all multipurpose facilities have fitness areas, gymnasiums, and a pool at a minimum. Racquet courts and tennis courts are less common features for most multipurpose clubs. Some multipurpose facilities also have outdoor facilities, such as outdoor pools, ball fields, and even team-building venues. The largest multipurpose clubs tend to be those that have tennis facilities, gymnasiums, and outdoor facilities. More often than not, multipurpose facilities tend to be located in suburban settings because of the space demands of such facilities and the lower cost of available land.

Health/fitness facilities come in an array of sizes, shapes, and designs. Some are quite large, while others are considerably smaller. Some conduct their operations on a single floor, while others occupy multiple floors. Some have a bland appearance externally as well as internally, while others feature a design concept that emphasizes a more polished "high-end" look.

Regardless of how large a facility is or how it looks, the key issue for a health/fitness facility is whether it is able to serve its intended and actual audience safely and effectively. This chapter addresses the factors in design and construction that can have a major impact on the ability of a health/fitness facility to provide a safe physical activity environment for its members and users.

Design and construction factors can be influenced by a number of considerations, including existing laws and regulations, architectural vision, available resources, and the activities and programs that are offered within a given facility. While some of these considerations are absolute in nature, others are not. For example, a facility's program offerings and certain design factors often go hand in hand. On one hand, the program offerings that are planned for a particular facility can have an influence on many of the decisions that are made concerning the design of a facility. On the other hand, the existing layout or space limitations within a given facility can help dictate (to a degree) what activity offerings are planned for that facility. Nonetheless, a health/fitness facility's program offerings typically play a key role in the level of success achieved by that facility.

This chapter presents standards and guidelines on health/fitness facility design and construction as they pertain to helping promote a safe physical activity environment for facility users. Table 6.1 details the two required standards in this regard, whereas table 6.2 lists the 11 recommended guidelines for health/fitness facility design and construction. This chapter is not intended as a comprehensive resource on health/fitness facility design and construction factors, but rather as a basic template for the design and construction features that are necessary for providing a reasonably safe physical activity environment.

TABLE 6.1   Standards for Health/Fitness Facility Design and Construction

1. Facilities, to the extent required by law, must adhere to the standards of building design that relate to the designing, building, expanding, or renovating of space as detailed in the Americans with Disabilities Act (ADA).

2. Facilities must be in compliance with all federal, state, and local building codes.

Health/fitness facility design and construction standard 1. Facilities, to the extent required by law, must adhere to the standards of building design that relate to the designing, building, expanding, or renovating of space as detailed in the Americans with Disabilities Act (ADA).

The ADA has established clear requirements for making facilities accessible to people with disabilities. In most instances, when a facility undergoes significant renovation or expansion or when a new facility is built, the ADA requires that the space be made accessible to people with disabilities. Depending on the extent of work being performed or the costs involved, there are instances in which a facility may be able to perform work without having to comply fully with the requirements of the ADA. Local building departments in most communities can assist facilities in obtaining a clearer understanding of the ADA requirements. Appendixes D and E provide additional details on accessibility requirements. Among the key elements that address accessibility within a health/fitness facility are the following:

- **Elevation changes.** The ADA requires that any change in elevation in excess of 0.5 in. (1.3 cm) must have a ramp or lift, with a slope of 12 in. (30 cm) for every inch in elevation change. A mechanical lift or elevator can be used in place of a ramp in cases of extreme changes in height.

- **Passageway width.** The ADA requires that doors, entryways, and exits have a width of at least 36 in. (91 cm) to accommodate wheelchair access. In addition, hallways and circulation passages need to have a width of at least 60 in. (152 cm).

- **Height of switches and fountains.** The ADA requires that all light switches, water fountains, fire extinguishers, and AED devices be at a height that can be reached by a user in a wheelchair.

- **Signage.** The ADA expects facilities to provide essential signage that can be viewed by those individuals who are visually impaired, particularly signage on emergency exits and signage that identifies other key space locations.

- **Clear floor space.** The ADA requires that each piece of equipment must have an adjacent clear floor space of at least 30 in. by 48 in. (76 cm by 122 cm).

Health/fitness facility design and construction standard 2. Facilities must be in compliance with all federal, state, and local building codes.

While federal requirements are consistent from one municipality to another, local building codes can vary drastically. Accordingly, it is imperative that facility operators be aware of the building codes in their community.

Standards for Health/Fitness Facility Design and Construction

TABLE 6.2	Guidelines for Health/Fitness Facility Design and Construction

1. Designers should size both physical activity spaces and nonactivity spaces to provide sufficient space to accommodate the expected user demand.

2. Designers should configure physical activity space plans so that defined circulation routes are adjacent to, rather than through, the various activity zones.

3. Facilities should provide open-access circulation, which avoids blind corners, unnecessary doors, partitions, and other hazards that would present a safety risk to members and users.

4. Designers should separate physical activity spaces from operational, storage, and maintenance spaces.

5. Facilities should provide all physical activity spaces with sufficient air circulation and fresh makeup air (i.e., outside air) to maintain air quality, room temperatures, and humidity at safe and comfortable levels. Notable exceptions to this particular guideline include such spaces as saunas, steam rooms, and hot yoga studios. However, even in these particular areas, measures to ensure safe and healthy human occupancy must be understood and implemented.

6. Facilities should illuminate all facility spaces to allow members and users to safely engage in their physical activity regimens. Minimum safe illumination levels vary according to activity in a particular area and should be carefully researched. The emerging need for energy conservation requires lighting solutions that take advantage of the available daylighting sources, automatic control devices, and the latest technologies in lamp and fixture design.

7. Facilities should be designed to maintain background noise levels below 70 decibels and never above 90 decibels. Sound transmission through defining perimeter partitions of a noise-generating activity area should be limited to a level that does not adversely affect the functionality level of neighboring spaces.

8. Floor surfaces in physical activity areas should meet specifications regarding the proper level of absorption and slip resistance to minimize the risk of fall-related injuries.

9. Facilities should have wall surfaces in activity spaces that are nonabrasive, flush, and free of protrusions that could cause impact injuries. Activity spaces that involve airborne projectiles, such as volleyballs or basketballs, should have a perimeter ball-containment barrier to protect users in adjacent areas and walkways.

10. When physical activity spaces have depth and distance parameters that can affect an individual's safety, then the facility should provide appropriate markings to ensure that users are aware of these depth and distance parameters.

11. Facilities should use "green" design and sustainable construction materials and techniques. Regardless of whether official certification is a desired goal, the widely published principles of green design related to site development, storm-water management, energy conservation, renewable resources, water conservation, indoor air quality, carbon reduction, and pollution control should be honored, whenever possible.

Health/fitness facility design and construction guideline 1. Designers should size both physical activity spaces and nonactivity spaces to provide sufficient space to accommodate the expected user demand.

While no standard metric is advocated for the allocation of health/fitness facility space per member, general industry statistics (based on *IHRSA's 2010 Profiles of Success*) show industry member occupancy levels (square feet per member or members per square foot) range from 10 sq ft (0.9 sq m) to 14 sq ft (1.3 sq m) per member. Empirical data from health/fitness operators around the globe show a general range of 0.3 sq m (3 sq ft) per member to 2.5 sq m (27 sq ft) per member. The allocation of space per member depends on the particular business model that a health/fitness facility operator chooses to adopt.

As for the allocation of space for a defined user or a defined piece of equipment in a fitness center, industry practice is to allocate approximately 40 to 60 sq ft (3.7 to 5.6 sq m) per piece of equipment in a fitness center or per user in a group exercise studio.

Health/fitness facility design and construction guideline 2. Designers should configure physical activity space plans so that defined circulation routes are adjacent to, rather than through, the various activity zones.

Circulation areas are spaces that allow users to enter, exit, and traverse the various physical activity zones. These circulation spaces are pathways that accommodate access to each area,* including the functional spaces in and around exercise equipment. To this end, circulation routes should be at least 36 in. (91 cm) across and should be located adjacent to the physical activity areas so that users do not have to pass directly through a physical activity area to access another area.

* *Note:* The ADA requires that one piece of each type of exercise equipment have a clear floor space equal to 30 in. by 48 in. (76 cm by 122 cm) and be served by an accessible route.

Health/fitness facility design and construction guideline 3. Facilities should provide open-access circulation, which avoids blind corners, unnecessary doors, partitions, and other hazards that would present a safety risk to members and users.

Open-access circulation refers to spaces that provide adequate sight lines and convenient access and egress for routine daily use and clear exit pathways during emergency situations. The following are some of the steps that a facility can take to provide open-access circulation:

- **Avoid blind corners in two-way circulation areas.** This objective can be accomplished in several ways, including soft corners, low walls at intersections, mirrors, and appropriate warning signage.

- **Avoid the use of doors that open up into circulation paths and hallways.** When doors are mandated by local codes or privacy situations, providing proper warning signage can help reduce any risk presented by these door locations.

- **Provide circulation areas that, by the nature of their design, communicate a path of safe passage.**

Health/fitness facility design and construction guideline 4. Designers should separate physical activity spaces from operational, storage, and maintenance spaces.

By separating back-of-the house operational spaces from physical activity spaces designed to be used by members and users, the designer can reduce or eliminate the likelihood that members and users will enter a facility area that would immediately expose them to an increased safety risk from items such as cleaning supplies, maintenance equipment, and related materials. The following are examples of back-of-the house operational areas that should be separated from the physical activity areas:

- **Laundry.** This area normally contains cleaning agents that, according to OSHA, present an increased risk of exposure to hazardous chemicals.

- **Equipment rooms for pools and whirlpools.** These areas commonly house chemicals and other agents that may be harmful, especially if inhaled directly.

- **Maintenance rooms.** These rooms commonly contain equipment (such as saws, chemical supplies, and power tools) that could accidentally cause harm to a facility member or user.

- **Mechanical and electrical rooms.** These rooms contain equipment that could expose members and users directly or indirectly to dangerous situations, such as exposed wires, high temperatures, and dangerous gases.

Health/fitness facility design and construction guideline 5. Facilities should provide all physical activity spaces with sufficient air circulation and fresh makeup air (i.e., outside air) to maintain air quality, room temperatures, and humidity at safe and comfortable levels. Notable exceptions to this particular guideline include such spaces as saunas, steam rooms, and hot yoga studios. However, even in these particular areas, measures to ensure safe and healthy human occupancy must be understood and implemented.

Air circulation is one of the most critical elements when designing and operating a health/fitness facility. When a room is filled with members and users exercising at a moderate to high level of intensity, the heat and humidity load increases dramatically. This situation can place an increased level of heat stress on the members and users and may result in dehydration, heat exhaustion, heatstroke, or (in rare instances) cardiovascular emergencies. In addition to the increased heat load that can result from improper air circulation, a risk of poor air quality exists that can expose members and users to airborne pathogens that can increase the risk of respiratory disorders or other airborne illnesses. Facilities can provide sufficient air circulation by taking into consideration the following factors:

- **Maintain relative humidity at 60% or lower in all physical activity spaces.** Ideally, a relative humidity level of 50% or lower is the desired goal, but maintaining levels below 60% is necessary.

- **Maintain air temperature for all physical activity areas between 68 and 72 °F (20 and 22 °C).** The key is to maintain these temperature ranges, whether the room is empty or fully occupied by members and users who are engaging in moderate to vigorous physical activity. This guideline refers to the fact that the heating, ventilation, and air conditioning (HVAC) system within the facility should have the capability to adjust airflow to meet the demands of each space. Ideally, a facility should be engineered with specific HVAC zones that can be individually controlled for a particular area, such as group activity studios, the fitness floor, racquet courts, locker rooms, pools, and wet areas.

- **Make sure that an adequate mix of external fresh air and recirculated internal air is moving through the facility.** The higher the percentage of external air, the less likely the chance that the system will circulate air that contains internally generated airborne pathogens or toxic out-gassing. The minimum level of outside external air is determined by building codes and is related to the specific use of the space.

- **Ensure that wet areas, such as shower areas, steam rooms, whirlpool areas, and swimming pools, have negative exhaust (more exhausted air than supplied air).** Negative pressure in wet areas allows air to be pulled from adjacent spaces rather than pushing damp and/or chlorine-scented air into these adjacent spaces.

- **Design engineers must make sure that the HVAC system is tested and balanced to provide air circulation at the proper volume (cubic feet per minute—CFM) and temperature in each physical activity area.** CFM is a quantitative measure that can be used to indicate the amount of airflow that is moved through a vent and into or out of a room. The CFM supplied for physical activity areas will vary based on the heat and occupant loads to which the area is exposed. For example, rooms, such as group exercise studios, will require higher CFM than racquet courts. Likewise, the cardiovascular equipment area will require higher CFM than the free weight area. Facilities should hire a qualified mechanical engineer to provide the specific system sizing and operational modes that are required in this regard. The proper balance of air circulation can ensure that all facility spaces are maintained at the intended temperature and humidity levels.

- **Keep the mechanical system clean.** Most mechanical systems require that the airstream be filtered and that these filters be cleaned or replaced on a prescribed and regular basis. This preventive maintenance will allow the system to provide better air circulation and will also prevent the buildup of dirt and microbes in the system.

Health/fitness facility design and construction guideline 6. Facilities should illuminate all facility spaces to allow members and users to safely engage in their physical activity regimens. Minimum safe illumination levels vary according to activity in a particular area and should be carefully researched. The emerging need for energy conservation requires lighting solutions that take advantage of the available daylighting sources, automatic control devices, and the latest technologies in lamp and fixture design.

Proper illumination is a necessity for a reasonably safe environment. The proper level of illumination can vary from space to space depending on the activity being performed. Spaces in which physical activity requires fine eye–hand motor coordination (e.g., playing tennis) require a higher degree of illumination compared with those facility areas (such as a yoga studio or massage room) where the need for lower levels of illumination might exist. Another important factor regarding proper levels of illumination is that a facility's users must be able to read all signage. The following are among the more important considerations for illumination:

- **Light levels in the majority of physical activity spaces, as measured at eye level, should be at least 50 foot-candles.** In selected areas, such as a tennis court or racquet court, light levels approaching 75 foot-candles at eye level are preferred, while on a volleyball court at floor level, a foot-candle level of 50 is appropriate. Each activity area will have slightly different illumination requirements based on the activity being performed. Lighting standards for most sporting activities are usually published by the relevant national association responsible for competitive standards.

- **When specifying light sources, an effort should be made to use light sources that are configured to produce soft, indirect lighting instead of direct lighting.** Natural lighting can be emphasized by using windows with tinted and insulated glass. Indirect light sources that bounce light off walls, floors, or ceilings are preferred to direct light sources, which often produce glare. The most often used, but least energy efficient, artificial lighting sources are incandescent lamps. Greater energy efficiency can be achieved with fluorescent light fixtures, compact fluorescent bulbs, metal-halide light fixtures, and mercury-vapor light fixtures.

- **Adjustable light sources (by means of multilevel switching or dimmers) should be provided, whenever possible, for areas such as group exercise studios, massage rooms, mind–body program areas, and similar spaces.** In certain spaces, such as group exercise studios, massage rooms, and yoga studios, variable lighting levels play an important role in establishing the type of environment conducive to the activity being housed. For example, in studios that serve multiple functions, such as a high-intensity group exercise class or a mind–body class, there is a need to adjust lighting levels to create the proper environment.

Health/fitness facility design and construction guideline 7. Facilities should be designed to maintain background noise levels below 70 decibels and never above 90 decibels. Sound transmission through defining perimeter partitions of a noise-generating activity area should be limited to a level that does not adversely affect the functionality level of neighboring spaces.

A health/fitness facility can be a cauldron of sounds, ranging from the background noise of members and users talking to the sound produced by audio systems. Noise levels are measured in decibels. Levels of 90 decibels or greater, regardless of circumstances, are too loud. Ongoing exposure of members, users, and staff to sound levels in excess of 90 decibels has been shown to cause hearing damage. Some health and fitness spaces, such as group exercise studios and the fitness floor, will naturally have higher decibel levels, while spaces such as the mind–body studio or the massage room generally have much lower decibel levels. As a general rule, decibel levels in the range of 30 to 40 allow for most individuals to receive sound without being exposed to noise levels that can result in damage to their hearing. Among the factors that should be taken into consideration when attempting to limit excessive decibel levels in a health/fitness facility are the following:

- **Group exercise studios tend to generate the highest decibel levels (levels between 80 and 90 decibels are common).** To assist in reducing the sound levels in these spaces, facilities should provide ceiling, floor, and wall surfaces that allow for moderate to excellent sound absorption; adjust audio systems so sound levels cannot be raised above 90 decibels; and develop and enforce policies that ensure that the facility's instructors adhere to the recommended sound levels. In addition, these spaces should be designed with additional sound-absorbing materials to prevent the movement of excess noise into adjacent spaces.

- **Spaces that require low levels of ambient noise (such as massage rooms, mind–body studios, and lounges) should be designed to have additional sound-absorbing materials in the ceilings, floors, and walls.** Impact sounds and vibrations are the most difficult noise to contain. The best way to prevent transmission of impact sounds is to mute them at their source by means of resilient surface materials before they can get into the building structure.

Health/fitness facility design and construction guideline 8. Floor surfaces in physical activity areas should meet specifications regarding the proper level of absorption and slip resistance to minimize the risk of fall-related injuries.

Some physical activity areas (such as the group exercise studio, basketball courts, racquet courts, sports courts, and the fitness floor) house activities that can expose users to impact stresses. In many cases, the activities performed in these areas can more than double the forces to which a member's or user's body is exposed. Fortunately, through the proper design and installation of floor surfaces, many of these additional forces can be absorbed by the floor surface rather than by the individual's musculoskeletal system. The key point with regard to floor surfaces is that facilities should adhere to the Deutsches Institut für Normung (DIN) standards when installing physical activity floor surfaces (see more details on page 90 in appendix B). According to the DIN standards, a floor must meet six criteria: shock absorption, standard vertical deflection, deflective indentation, sliding characteristics, ball deflection, and rolling load. Each of these six characteristics can be used to help evaluate the suitability of a floor for specific physical activity functions, including the following:

- **Sport function.** These are floors that serve a recreational or performance sport function, such as a basketball court or racquetball court. These court floors need to provide good surface friction and ball reflection. In deciding which floors to use for this purpose, it is critical to employ a consistent subfloor that absorbs impact equally at all points on the floor and generates minimal deflective indentation. In addition, these floors should provide a moderate level of surface friction that balances the ability to gain traction with the ability for sliding. These floors normally have a subfloor system (consisting of furring strips and shock-absorbing materials) that is covered by a solid wood surface or a rubber surface that allows for sliding movement.

- **Protective function.** The primary role served by these floors is the reduction of chronic-impact injuries or acute-impact injuries, such as those that could occur in a group exercise studio. These floors should have an appropriate level of shock absorption, minimal vertical deformation, and expose participants to an appropriate level of friction. Normally, these floors have a three-layer system, consisting of a bottom shock-absorbing layer (neoprene shock pads, rubber pads, springs), a middle layer that has multiple layers of plywood, and a top layer consisting of a wood or rubber surface.

- **Material–technical function.** These floors, which should meet criteria for both sport and protective function, are excellent for facilities that use space for multiple activities, such as a basketball court that also serves as a group exercise space. According to the DIN standards, this type of floor should have the following characteristics:

Shock absorption	53%
Minimum vertical deformation	2.3 mm
Minimum deflective indentation	15%
Maximum sliding characteristic	0.5 to 0.7 range
Ball deflection	90% minimum
Rolling load	337.6 lb (153.1 kg)

Facility operators should discuss their facility's requirements with floor manufacturers to ensure that the floors that they select for their facility are constructed in accordance with DIN standards.

Health/fitness facility design and construction guideline 9. Facilities should have wall surfaces in activity spaces that are nonabrasive, flush, and free of protrusions that could cause impact injuries. Activity spaces that involve airborne projectiles, such as volleyballs and basketballs, should have a perimeter ball-containment barrier to protect individuals in adjacent areas and walkways.

A designer should make sure that walls in activity areas don't contain protrusions (e.g., a railing that protrudes onto a court surface, a storage shelf that extends into the activity area of a group exercise studio) that might result in a member or user accidently making contact with the protrusion while engaging in a physical activity regimen.

Health/fitness facility design and construction guideline 10. When physical activity spaces have depth and distance parameters that can affect an individual's safety, then the facility should provide appropriate markings to ensure that users are aware of these depth and distance parameters.

Certain physical activity areas, such as pools, gymnasiums (sports courts), and racquet courts, have depth and distance parameters that can result in a potential injury if members and users are unaware of them. As a result, it is advisable to provide markings so that members and users can easily differentiate specific changes in depth or distance without incurring bodily harm. Examples of markings include the following:

- **Pools.** Pools present the greatest risk to member and user safety because of the presence of water and changes in depth. Facilities should follow the parameters developed by the National Spa and Pool Institute (NSPI) for marking pool depths and distances, subject to local and state codes. Pools are expected to provide proper depth markings at various points, especially when there are changes in pool depth.

- **Basketball courts and racquetball courts.** These courts have specific markings and dimensions established by the respective sport governing bodies. Facilities should ensure that these recommendations are followed in the design and installation of the courts.

- **Walking and jogging tracks.** These are another facility component where adequate dimensions must be provided. Lane widths and designations for walkers and runners are important. Care must be exercised to avoid blind corners and potential trip-and-fall hazards resulting from inadequate clearances from columns, rails, and walls adjacent to the running lanes.

Additional details on specific design or construction parameters for health/fitness facilities are presented in appendix B.

Health/fitness facility design and construction guideline 11. Facilities should use "green" design and sustainable construction materials and techniques. Regardless of whether official certification is a desired goal, the widely published principles of green design related to site development, storm-water management, energy conservation, renewable resources, water conservation, indoor air quality, carbon reduction, and pollution control should be honored, whenever possible.

Over the past five years, green design, also known as sustainable design, has become more prevalent in many industries, including the health/fitness industry. Green design refers to practices that make use of environmentally friendly materials (e.g., recycled glass, recycled rubber products, renewable wood products, naturally renewable products, low-volatility paint products) as well as renewable and efficient energy systems (e.g., solar-powered heating and lighting, reclaimed rainwater systems, low-energy lighting systems, geothermal heating). In addition to the aforementioned green design elements, using high-efficiency long-life lamp technologies, dual-flush toilets, low-flow shower heads, and so on, all contribute to a more efficient and sustainable environment for facility users. One means of achieving green design is to retain the services of an architect that is Leadership in Energy and Environmental Design (LEED) certified. Green design not only contributes to a healthy planet but also provides users of a fitness facility with a healthier environment for their physical activity efforts.

CHAPTER 7

Health/Fitness Facility Equipment

According to empirical data from the health/fitness facility industry, a typical health/ fitness facility will invest between $20 and $25 per square foot ($215 to $270 per square meter) on fitness equipment before opening its doors to the public for the first time. This relatively large investment indicates the important role that fitness equipment plays in providing facility users with the opportunity to pursue their physical activity interests and needs. This initial investment in equipment is further compounded by the need for facility owners to reinvest in equipment on an annual basis to stay current with equipment trends (entertainment, function, and safety) and to deal with the depreciation and inevitable wear on fitness equipment. According to *IHRSA's 2010 Profiles of Success*, the median reinvestment allocation for fitness equipment in health/fitness facilities in 2009 was 1.3% of revenues, with some health/facility operators allocating as much as 4.7% of revenues on an annual basis to reinvesting in fitness equipment.

The basic categories of fitness equipment that play the most significant role in the industry when it comes to delivering physical activity programs are cardiovascular equipment, variable-resistance and selectorized resistance equipment, free weight equipment, and fitness accessory equipment.

- **Cardiovascular equipment.** According to *IHRSA's 2010 Profiles of Success*, five of the top six usage areas of a health/fitness facility involve cardiovascular equipment (treadmills offered by 64% of facilities, elliptical trainers offered by 62% of facilities, recumbent bikes offered by 62% of facilities, and upright bikes offered by 62% of facilities). Cardiovascular equipment consistently ranks as one of the top areas of equipment reinvestment for facility operators. Although cardiovascular equipment has been around for almost as long as the health and fitness industry has been in existence, over the last 15 years, it has taken on an escalating level of importance in the marketing and programming of health/fitness facilities.

- **Variable-resistance and selectorized resistance equipment.** According to statistics provided by IHRSA, variable-resistance (rank 26th) and selectorized resistance (rank 11th) equipment rank just behind cardiovascular equipment in terms of importance (ranks according to *2010 Profiles of Success*). Selectorized resistance equipment is strength training equipment that uses weight stacks and pulley mechanisms to provide resistance. The advantage of this type of resistance exercise is that it provides a safe and time-efficient method of strength training, one that often has particular appeal for the average health/

fitness facility member or user. Variable-resistance equipment is quite similar to selectorized resistance equipment except that it employs a device (usually a cam) that allows the level of resistance provided to the exerciser at any given point in time to vary according to predetermined strength curve of the muscles involved in the exercise.

- **Free weight equipment.** Free weight equipment has been in existence longer than any other form of exercise equipment, dating back to the 1800s. According to *IHRSA's 2010 Profiles of Success*, free weight equipment was offered by more than 83% of the clubs surveyed. This statistic, one that continues from year to year in the annual IIRSA survey, indicates that free weight equipment remains one of the most popular types of fitness equipment in the health and fitness club industry.

- **Fitness accessory equipment.** Fitness accessory equipment includes Pilates gear, bands and tubes, fitness-testing apparatus, plyometric paraphernalia, medicine balls, exercise balls, kettlebells, foam rollers, and other devices that can assist individuals in achieving their health and fitness goals. Additional fitness accessories that are often found in health/fitness facilities include equipment (such as weight training belts and protective lenses) that can be used to provide a safer environment for a facility's members and users as they engage in activities of their choosing.

This chapter presents standards and guidelines pertaining to equipment that is found in health/fitness facilities. Table 7.1 details the one required standard on health/fitness facility equipment; table 7.2 lists the five recommended guidelines that health/fitness facilities should consider when acquiring fitness equipment. The chapter also contains tables 7.3 and 7.4 which address general preventive maintenance practices that facility operators can take with resistance training and cardiovascular equipment. It should be noted that this chapter is not intended to provide an in-depth review of health and fitness equipment. Rather, it is designed to offer information regarding equipment that health/fitness facilities can use in their efforts to provide a safe and productive physical activity environment for their members and users.

TABLE 7.1 **Standards for Health/Fitness Facility Equipment**
1. The aquatic and pool facilities must provide the proper safety equipment according to state and local codes and regulations.

Health/fitness facility equipment standard 1. The aquatic and pool facilities must provide the proper safety equipment according to state and local codes and regulations.

State and local governments have specific requirements regarding the safety equipment that must be present in an aquatic area. Examples of the types of equipment that may be required include a spine board, a 25 ft (7.6 m) safety rope with a buoy, a shepherd's crook, lifejackets, a rescue tube, blankets, and a first-aid kit. If a facility has more than one aquatic venue, each venue must have the proper equipment.

TABLE 7.2 Guidelines for Health/Fitness Facility Equipment

1. Facility operators should provide a sufficient quantity and quality of equipment so that the facility is able to fulfill its mission, purpose, and intended function for its targeted members and users.
2. Facility operators should have a preventive maintenance program for their fitness equipment, including documentation showing when the scheduled work was performed.
3. Facility operators should have a system in place for removing broken or damaged equipment from member use until that equipment has been repaired or replaced.
4. All physical activity areas should have a clock, a chart of target heart rates, and a chart depicting ratings of perceived exertion to enable members and users to monitor their level of physical exertion.
5. Facility operators should consider providing a few pieces of fitness equipment that can be accessed by individuals with physical limitations who require the use of a wheelchair, including at least one piece of cardiovascular equipment and one piece of selectorized or variable-resistance equipment.

Health/fitness facility equipment guideline 1. Facility operators should provide a sufficient quantity and quality of equipment so that the facility is able to adequately fulfill its mission, purpose, and intended function for its targeted members and users.

Health/fitness facilities vary considerably in their intended mission and purpose. For example, some facilities, such as multipurpose facilities, focus on serving the fitness and recreational needs of the family market, while fitness-only clubs address the muscular strength and endurance interests of a young male population. In recent years, a substantial number of women-only facilities have opened; their basic business model involves providing a nonintimidating general fitness environment for their clients. Such diversity of missions and purposes has a significant impact on the variety, quantity, and quality of equipment that is made available to members and users.

Decisions concerning the kind of equipment to buy, how much equipment to buy, and how much to spend on equipment can be affected by a number of factors, which can vary from facility to facility. The following information can be used to help clarify the key issues pertaining to such discussions:

- **Cardiovascular equipment.** The second most popular category of equipment in the health and fitness industry, cardiovascular equipment should be part of every health/fitness facility. The most popular types of cardiovascular equipment include treadmills, elliptical trainers, recumbent bicycles, upright bicycles, rowing machines, stair climbers, upper-body ergometers, and total-body machines (e.g., cross-body trainers). Health/fitness facilities should consider offering at least three types of cardiovascular equipment (e.g., treadmills, elliptical trainers, and bicycles). The minimum number of pieces for a specific type of cardiovascular equipment should be two machines; the ideal quantity is dependent on variables such as the number of members, expected usage during peak periods, member demographics, and so on.

While no precise criteria exist in the industry for determining the appropriate quantity or mix of cardiovascular equipment, common practice in the industry is to provide sufficient equipment to accommodate at least 25% of the individuals who are expected to use the facility during any given two-hour time period. For example, if a hypothetical facility has 2,000 members and users, then that facility is likely to see approximately 500 (or 25%) of those members on a daily basis. Furthermore, during any given two-hour time period, it can expect to see no more than 33% of those daily users, or 165 users. If the criterion is one piece of cardiovascular equipment for every 4 members and users in a facility, then the facility in this example would need approximately 40 pieces of cardiovascular equipment.

- **Variable-resistance and selectorized resistance equipment.** Variable-resistance and selectorized resistance machines are designed to provide individuals with a relatively safe, time-efficient method to engage in strength exercise. Some of these machines have multiple stations that collectively offer a whole-body workout. Others address only a single muscle or area of the body. In those instances, a series of selectorized resistance and/or variable-resistance machines will be required for achieving a complete strength training regimen. At a minimum, one machine for each major muscle group in the body will be required. Depending on the facility's organizational focus, it is recommended that every health/fitness facility have at least one resistance circuit (typically 8 to 12 machines). At a minimum, health/fitness facilities should make sure that they have sufficient machines to accommodate anticipated demand by its members and users for strength exercise. While no specific industry criteria exist in this regard, common practice within the health/fitness industry dictates that at least one circuit should be provided for each 1,000 members and users.

- **Free weight equipment.** The most popular type of exercise equipment in health/fitness facilities is free weight equipment, which can include such items as dumbbells, barbells and plates, plate-loaded benches and machines, and benches and machines that can be used for performing exercises that employ barbells and dumbbells. The type and quantity of free weight equipment that a facility provides will depend on that facility's membership and usage patterns as well as its targeted audience.

- **Fitness accessory equipment.** Over the past 10 years, the interest in and the demand for functional and performance-based fitness training have grown tremendously. Types of fitness accessory equipment that can facilitate such functional and performance-based training include, but are not limited to, medicine balls, exercise balls, tubes and bands, foam rollers, kettlebells, BOSU balls, Pilates-based equipment, plyometric benches, rope ladders, cones, and steps. The quantity of fitness accessory equipment that a facility acquires is highly dependent on the facility's member and user demographics, the number of facility members and users, and the qualifications of its staff and independent contractors.

- **Group exercise equipment.** Group exercise studios are one of the most highly used spaces in a health/fitness facility. The types of program offerings that are typically conducted in a group exercise area include, but are not limited to, group cycling classes, stretching classes, low-impact classes, yoga classes, martial arts fitness classes, callisthenic classes, weight equipment–based classes, and sport performance classes. Because of the large variety of classes that can be offered within such areas, a facility should provide the equipment that is necessary to accommodate the needs of those classes. Ancillary group exercise equipment for these classes may include group cycles, exercise mats, step benches, tubes and bands, exercise balls, body bars, dumbbells, and medicine balls.

Health/fitness facility equipment guideline 2. Facilities should have a preventive maintenance program for their fitness equipment, including documentation showing when the scheduled work was performed.

Manufacturers of fitness equipment provide limited warranties on their equipment as well as recommendations for its ongoing care. The proper care of equipment is essential for several reasons. For example, failure to have and adhere to a preventive maintenance system will almost always lead to equipment breakdowns and a heightened risk to users' safety and the facility's subsequent exposure to litigation. In most instances, the preventive maintenance of fitness equipment is quite straightforward. As a rule, facilities, are encouraged to closely follow the manufacturer's recommendations for standard preventive maintenance. Tables 7.3 and 7.4 provide an overview of the most common preventive maintenance practices for resistance equipment and cardiovascular equipment, respectively.

TABLE 7.3 Common Preventive Maintenance Practices for Resistance Equipment

Equipment	Daily	Weekly	Monthly	As needed
Variable-resistance equipment	• Clean frames with mild soap and water. • Clean upholstery with mild soap and water.	• Check all cables and bolts, and tighten as needed. • Check moving parts, and adjust as needed.	Lubricate guide rods with lightweight oil.	• Repair or replace pads. • Replace cables if needed.
Free weight benches	• Clean frames with mild soap and water. • Clean upholstery with mild soap and water.	• Check all cables and bolts, and tighten as needed. • Check moving parts, and adjust as needed.		• Repair or replace pads. • Replace cables if needed.
Dumbbells and bars	Clean off bars with dry cloth.	Check all screws and bolts, and tighten as needed.	Use lightweight oil on cloth to remove any rust.	Repair or replace broken bars and dumbbells.

TABLE 7.4 Common Preventive Maintenance Practices for Cardiovascular Equipment

Equipment	Daily	Weekly	Monthly	As needed
Bikes	• Clean off control panel with dry cloth. • Clean off handles with mild antibacterial soap and damp cloth. • Clean off seats with mild antibacterial soap and damp cloth.	• Check equipment diagnostics through control panel for any potential troubles. • Check all screws and bolts, and tighten as needed.	Remove bike housing, and clean out dust and lint that may have collected.	Refer to manufacturer's guidelines.
Elliptical trainers	• Clean off control panel with dry cloth. • Clean off handles with mild antibacterial soap and damp cloth. • Clean off foot pedals with damp cloth.	• Check equipment diagnostics through control panel for any potential troubles. • Check all screws and bolts, and tighten as needed.	Remove elliptical housing, and clean out dust and lint that may have collected.	Refer to manufacturer's guidelines.
Treadmills	• Clean off control panels with dry cloth. • Clean off housing with mild antibacterial soap and damp cloth.	• Check equipment diagnostics through control panel for any potential troubles. • Check all screws and bolts, and tighten as needed.	• Clean belt using a damp cloth. • Check belt and deck surface, and lubricate as needed and per manufacturer's specifications.	• Replace belt if needed. • Refer to manufacturer's guidelines.

Guidelines for Health/Fitness Facility Equipment

Health/fitness facility equipment guideline 3. Facility operators should have a system in place for removing broken or damaged equipment from member use until that equipment has been repaired or replaced.

Fitness equipment that is either broken or damaged can pose a risk to the safety of members and users. As a result, facility operators should establish polices to address the removal of broken and/or damaged equipment from areas where it can be used by members and users, until such time as it is repaired or replaced by a newly functioning piece. These polices should include a transparent approach to communicating to the members and users that a piece of equipment is temporarily damaged and out of order, along with communication as to when the piece will be repaired or replaced.

Health/fitness facility equipment guideline 4. All physical activity areas should have a clock, a chart of target heart rates, and a chart depicting ratings of perceived exertion to enable members and users to monitor their level of physical exertion.

Health/fitness facility operators should have a clock and a target heart rate chart available in various physical activity areas (e.g., cardiovascular zone, variable-resistance zone, group exercise studio) to allow facility members and users to monitor their level of physical exertion and assist them in achieving their desired training intensity and duration. A ratings of perceived exertion chart can be substituted for or used to complement a target heart rate chart as a means of providing individuals with an easy-to-understand method of monitoring their level of intensity of physical activity.

Health/fitness facility equipment guideline 5. Facility operators should consider providing a few pieces of fitness equipment that can be accessed by individuals with physical limitations who require the use of a wheelchair, including at least one piece of cardiovascular equipment and one piece of selectorized or variable-resistance equipment.

Individuals with physical limitations who require the use of a wheelchair or other mobility device can receive the same health benefits from exercise as individuals who do not have physical limitations. As a result, health/fitness operators should make an effort to provide this group of members and users with access to fitness equipment. Typically, this factor might involve providing at least one piece of cardiovascular equipment, such as an upper-body ergometer or a cross-functional piece, that provides those individuals who are unable to use their legs with the ability to perform continuous cardiovascular movements. In addition, many manufacturers currently produce selectorized resistance machines that can be easily accessed by individuals in wheelchairs. As such, health/fitness facility operators should consider incorporating at least one of these units into their selectorized resistance selection.

CHAPTER 8

Signage in Health/ Fitness Facilities

Signage is one of the most important means by which health/fitness facilities communicate with their members and users and the general public. Signage can help convey a variety of messages, including hazard warnings, cautionary warnings, instructions on the proper use of a piece of equipment, and general facility information. When signage is developed and displayed properly, it allows the desired message to be communicated clearly and in a timely manner. On the other hand, poorly conceived and displayed signage can result in either confusion or a complete failure to communicate the desired message.

Signage can serve many communication roles in a health/fitness facility (e.g., providing physical directions for members and users, instructing on the safe and effective use of equipment, providing information about facility services, and warning about conditions in the facility that might expose members and users to unwarranted risk). Proper signage plays a critical role in establishing a safer physical activity environment. It should be noted, however, that no label or sign alone can prevent all injuries or ensure that all members and users engage in risk-free practices. In that regard, ASTM International (originally known as the American Society for Testing and Materials) developed and issued F1749, titled *Standard Specification for Fitness Equipment and Fitness Facility Safety Signage and Labels,* which sets forth guidelines for signage and labels associated with fitness equipment and fitness facilities that can promote a higher level of safety in a health/fitness facility.

This chapter presents standards and guidelines on signage and its use in a health/fitness facility. Table 8.1 lists the five required standards on signage in health/fitness facilities, and table 8.3 details the two recommended guidelines on signage in health/fitness facilities. This chapter also contains table 8.2 that sets forth some area-specific safety and warning messages that are frequently seen in a health/fitness facility.

TABLE 8.1 Standards for Signage in Health/Fitness Facilities

1. Facility operators shall post proper caution, danger, and warning signage in conspicuous locations where facility staff know, or should know, that existing conditions and situations warrant such signage.

2. Facility operators shall post the appropriate emergency and safety signage pertaining to fire and related emergency situations, as required by federal, state, and local codes.

3. Facility operators shall post signage indicating the location of any AED and first-aid kits, including directions on how to access those locations.

4. Facilities shall post all ADA and OSHA signage that is required by federal, state, and local laws and regulations.

5. All cautionary, danger, and warning signage shall have the required signal icon, signal word, signal color, and layout as specified in ASTM F1749.

Health/fitness facility signage standard 1. Facility operators shall post proper caution, danger, and warning signage in conspicuous locations where facility staff know, or should know, that existing conditions and situations warrant such signage.

A facility has the responsibility to provide members and users with information about conditions and situations that might expose them to an increased risk of experiencing an injury, a health-related problem, or even death. In that regard, the following three types of signage are appropriate:

- **Cautionary signage.** Cautionary signage is designed to alert members and users of the potential risks that exist or the hazardous situations that might arise from using a particular piece of equipment, from circumstances inherent in a given facility area, or from their participation in a specific program or service that is offered by the facility. Cautionary signage must provide members and users with both a cautionary statement and a concrete list of actions that are appropriate to avoid the risk(s) indicated in the cautionary statement.

- **Danger signage.** Danger signage is designed to provide members and users with a clear message that indicates that an *imminent* hazardous situation exists, and, if that situation is not avoided, serious injury or death may result. Danger signage must provide members and users with a clear statement of the applicable danger and what steps must be taken to avoid that danger or risk.

- **Warning signage.** Warning signage is designed to provide members and users with a clear message indicating that a *potentially* hazardous situation exists and, if it is not avoided, death or serious injury could occur. Warning signage should provide members and users with a clear statement that warns them of the potential risks that apply to a particular situation and the measures that can be taken to avoid the risks. Table 8.2 offers an example of a few area-specific safety and warning messages. In each situation, the basic objective of such signage is specified.

TABLE 8.2   Examples of Area-Specific Safety and Warning Signage

Activity area	Examples of safety warnings
Fitness floor (gym)	Exercising may cause conditions, such as dizziness, light-headedness, disorientation, exhaustion, or other signs or symptoms, that put the exerciser at risk. If you experience any of these warnings, you should cease exercising and contact a member of the staff.
	Please seek out the assistance of fitness professionals before beginning a fitness program.
	Heart rate charts and charts of perceived exertion are posted throughout the fitness area to assist you with monitoring your level of exertion during exercise.
Sauna or steam room	Users should limit themselves to no more than 10 minutes in the sauna to avoid the possibility of heat exhaustion or heatstroke.
	Members and users with cardiovascular disease, high blood pressure, or other medical conditions that could be exacerbated by exposure to high temperatures should consult a medical professional before entering the sauna.
Pool	Shower before entering the pool.
	Do not dive into the pool.
	A lifeguard is not on duty, and, therefore, swimming is taken at your own risk.

Health/fitness facility signage standard 2. Facility operators shall post the appropriate emergency and safety signage pertaining to fire and related emergency situations, as required by federal, state, and local codes.

It is imperative that facilities comply with all federal, state, and local laws when it comes to the posting of signage pertaining to fire and related emergency situations. As part of the process, it is recommended that all health/fitness facilities consult with both their local fire department and local city authorities to ensure that they are in full compliance with all fire safety and emergency signage. Factors that such signage must address may include the following:

- **Emergency exit signage.** These signs not only show the location of all emergency exits but also provide directions for how to proceed to these exits.

- **Emergency phone and fire extinguisher location signage.** These signs identify the location of telephones and fire extinguishers and provide instructions for their use.

- **Facility occupancy load and certificate of occupancy.** This signage indicates the maximum number of members and users who are allowed in the facility at any given time, according to local building codes.

Health/fitness facility signage standard 3. Facility operators shall post signage indicating the location of any AED and first-aid kits, including directions on how to access those locations.

Facility operators shall provide signs that identify the location of all AED units and first-aid kits. In addition to identifying the location of these devices, signage must clearly communicate directions on how to get to these locations.

Standards for Signage in Health/Fitness Facilities

Health/fitness facility signage standard 4. Facilities shall post all ADA and OSHA signage that is required by federal, state, and local laws and regulations.

Both the Americans with Disabilities Act (ADA) and the Occupational Safety and Health Administration (OSHA) provide explicit regulations regarding the posting of certain signage. For example, OSHA requires that a facility operator post warning signage for hazardous chemicals and blood-borne pathogens if the member or user may be exposed to either. The ADA expects facilities to provide signage that indicates access points for people with physical challenges, as well as certain signage that can be viewed by some individuals who have visual impairments.

Health/fitness facility signage standard 5. All cautionary, danger, and warning signage shall have the required signal icon, signal word, signal color, and layout as specified in ASTM F1749.

The standards and guidelines from both the American National Standards Institute (ANSI) and ASTM International spell out the specific parameters for appearance required for the design and layout of cautionary, danger, and warning signage, including the color of the sign, the wording to be provided, and the type of icon to be used.

TABLE 8.3	**Guidelines for Signage in Health/Fitness Facilities**

1. Facilities should provide message boards, bulletin boards, electronic bulletin boards, websites, or a similar type of communication venue for the communication and dissemination of relevant information on the facility or of particular interest to the facility's members.
2. Signage should have the proper appearance, readability, and placement in order to clearly display the desired message in a fashion that can easily be understood by the intended audience.

Health/fitness facility signage guideline 1. Facilities should provide message boards, bulletin boards, electronic bulletin boards, websites, or a similar type of communication venue for the communication and dissemination of relevant information on the facility or of particular interest to the facility's members.

To provide a safer and more enjoyable physical activity experience for members and users, facilities should post pertinent information on appropriate communication sites for members and users to access. A low-tech approach to such communication might involve bulletin boards or message boards that are positioned in highly visible locations throughout the facility. As technology has advanced, health/fitness facilities should seriously consider using their website, in-house electronic media centers, or even smart phone-based applications to disseminate relevant information to members and users. The type of information that should be communicated might include updates on facility programs and services, rules and policies of the facility, facts about certain staff members and their qualifications, and related information. The following examples illustrate the various types of information that this guideline could address:

- **Facility program calendars and schedules.** Facility operators can use these communication tools to share with members and users information about selected activities that will be offered during a specified time period. Examples of these types of tools include group exercise schedules, monthly program calendars, and special-event posters.

- **Facility policies and rules.** Facility operators can employ these communication tools to detail to their members and users the expectations of the facility concerning basic fundamental issues, such as operating hours, dress code, age restrictions, and appropriate behavior of users.

- **User comments and suggestions.** Facility operators can employ these communication tools as a means whereby members and users can be surveyed or as a way to post messages about their experiences in the facility or about services relating to the facility on which they would like to provide feedback.

- **Facility staff information.** Facilities can use these communication tools to share information with members and users about key staff and their qualifications. This mechanism can be an especially useful way to provide relevant information about personal trainers and other physical activity instructors.

Guidelines for Signage in Health/Fitness Facilities

Health/fitness facility signage guideline 2. Signage should have the proper appearance, readability, and placement in order to clearly display the desired message in a fashion that can easily be understood by the intended audience.

The following points delineate the relevant factors that a facility should consider regarding signage:

- **Appearance.** A sign should use colors and materials that are most likely to communicate the desired message. For instance, it is recommended that the color red be used for danger, orange for warning, and yellow for caution. The type of material used in the sign can also be important. For example, a waterproof material should be used for all signage that is posted in areas exposed to high humidity and water.

- **Readability.** This factor refers to the words, symbols, pictures, and typeface that are used to build the signage. For example, whenever possible, line drawings and illustrations should be used on signage, since they often have universal meaning. Moreover, the use of certain symbols, such as a person falling, can indicate that a condition exists that presents a slip-and-fall danger. Any typeface used on the signage should be bold and large enough so that the reader can easily read the message from a distance.

- **Placement.** This feature refers to the location of signage. Signs should be placed in conspicuous locations that can be easily seen by the user. Signs should be placed at eye level and have sufficient white space or open space around them so that the reader's focus is clearly directed to the intended message of the signage.

Blueprint for Excellence

The primary purpose of this appendix is to provide a summary of the 34 standards and 37 guidelines that are detailed in chapters 1 through 8 of the book.

Collectively, these standards and guidelines are addressed in chapters 1 to 8, grouped and dealt with by topic (pre-activity screening; orientation, education, and supervision; risk management and emergency policies; professional staff and independent contractors; facility design and construction; equipment; operating practices; signage). Each chapter includes both an overview of the standards and guidelines attendant to a particular topic and a discussion of the rationale underlying each standard and guideline.

Table A.1 provides a list of the 34 standards and table A.2 provides a list of the 37 guidelines that appear in detail in chapters one through eight, and which have been identified as appropriate for health/fitness facilities. The chapter in which each standard and guideline is covered is noted in parentheses following each specific listing.

TABLE A.1 Standards for Health/Fitness Facilities

1. Facility operators shall offer a general pre-activity screening tool (e.g., Par-Q) and/or specific pre-activity screening tool (e.g., health risk appraisal [HRA], health history questionnaire [HHQ]) to all new members and prospective users (chapter 1).

2. General pre-activity screening tools (e.g., PAR-Q) shall provide an authenticated means for new members, and/or users to identify whether a level of risk exists that indicates that they should seek consultation from a qualified healthcare professional prior to engaging in a program of physical activity (chapter 1).

3. All specific pre-activity screening tools (e.g., HRA, HHQ) shall be reviewed and interpreted by qualified staff (e.g., a qualified health/fitness professional or healthcare professional), and the results of the review and interpretation shall be retained on file by the facility for a period of at least one year from the time the tool was reviewed and interpreted (chapter 1).

4. If a facility operator becomes aware that a member, user, or prospective user has a known cardiovascular, metabolic, or pulmonary disease, or two or more major cardiovascular disease risk factors, or any other self-disclosed medical concern, that individual shall be advised to consult with a qualified healthcare provider before beginning a physical activity program (chapter 1).

5. Facilities shall provide a means for communicating to existing members (e.g., those who have been members for greater than 90 days) the value of completing a general and/or specific pre-activity screening tool on a regular basis (e.g., preferably once annually) during the course of their membership. Such communication can be done through a variety of mechanisms, including but not limited to a statement incorporated into the membership agreement of the facility, a statement on the new-member pre-activity screening form, and a statement on the website (chapter 1).

6. Once a new member or prospective user has completed a pre-activity screening process, facility operators shall then offer the new member or prospective user a general orientation to the facility (chapter 2).

7. Facilities shall provide a means by which members and users who are engaged in a physical activity program within the facility can obtain assistance and/or guidance with their physical activity program (chapter 2).

8. Facility operators must have written emergency response policies and procedures, which shall be reviewed regularly and physically rehearsed at least twice annually. These policies shall enable staff to respond to basic first-aid situations and emergency events in an appropriate and timely manner (chapter 3).

9. Facility operators shall ensure that a safety audit is conducted that routinely inspects all areas of the facility to reduce or eliminate unsafe hazards that may cause injury to employees and health/fitness facility members or health/fitness facility users (chapter 3).

10. Facility operators shall have a written system for sharing information with members and users, employees, and independent contractors regarding the handling of potentially hazardous materials, including the handling of bodily fluids by the facility staff in accordance with the guidelines of the U.S. Occupational Safety and Health Administration (OSHA) (chapter 3).

11. In addition to complying with all applicable federal, state, and local requirements relating to automated external defibrillators (AEDs), all facilities (e.g., staffed or unstaffed) shall have as part of their written emergency response policies and procedures a public access defibrillation (PAD) program in accordance with generally accepted practice, as highlighted in this section (chapter 3).

12. AEDs in a facility shall be located within a 1.5-minute walk to any place an AED could be potentially needed (chapter 3).

13. A skills review, practice sessions, and a practice drill with the AED shall be conducted a minimum of every six months, covering a variety of potential emergency situations (e.g., water, presence of a pacemaker, medications, children) (chapter 3).

14. A staffed facility shall assign at least one staff member to be on duty during all facility operating hours who is currently trained and certified in the delivery of cardiopulmonary resuscitation and in the administration of an AED (chapter 3).

15. Unstaffed facilities must comply with all applicable federal, state, and local requirements relating to AEDs. Unstaffed facilities shall have as part of their written emergency response policies and procedures a PAD program as a means by which either members and users or an external emergency responder can respond from time of collapse to defibrillation in four minutes or less (chapter 3).

16. The health/fitness professionals who have supervisory responsibility and oversight responsibility for the physical activity programs and the staff who administer them shall have an appropriate level of professional education, work experience, and/or certification. Examples of health/fitness professionals who serve in a supervisory role include the fitness director, group exercise director, aquatics director, and program director (chapter 4).

17. The health/fitness and healthcare professionals who serve in counseling, instruction, and physical activity supervision roles for the facility shall have an appropriate level of professional education, work experience, and/or certification. The primary professional staff and independent contractors who serve in these roles are fitness instructors, group exercise instructors, lifestyle counselors, and personal trainers (chapter 4).

18. Health/fitness and healthcare professionals engaged in pre-activity screening or prescribing, instructing, monitoring, or supervising of physical activity programs for facility members and users shall have current automated external defibrillation and cardiopulmonary resuscitation (AED and CPR) certification from an organization qualified to provide such certification. A certification should include a practical examination (chapter 4).

19. Facilities shall have an operational system in place that monitors, either manually or technologically, the presence and identity of all individuals (e.g., members and users) who enter into and participate in the activities, programs, and services of the facility (chapter 5).

20. Facilities that offer a sauna, steam room, or whirlpool shall have a technical monitoring system in place to ensure that these areas are maintained at the proper temperature and humidity level and that the appropriate warning systems and signage are in place to notify members and users of any risks related to the use of these areas, including subsequent unsafe changes in temperature and humidity (chapter 5).

21. Facilities that offer members and users access to a pool or whirlpool shall provide evidence that they comply with all water-chemistry safety requirements mandated by state and local codes and regulations (chapter 5).

22. A facility that offers youth services or programs shall provide evidence that it complies with all applicable state and local laws and regulations pertaining to their supervision (chapter 5).

23. When a child is under direct staff supervision of a facility, as a participant in either an organized activity or in an ongoing facility program, or is just under temporary staff supervision while the parent or legal guardian is using the facility, the responsible staff person shall have ready access to the child's basic medical information, which has been previously collected from the parent as part of the child registration process (chapter 5).

24. The registration policy of a facility that provides child care shall require that parents or guardians of all children left in the facility's care complete a waiver, an authorization for emergency medical care, and a release for the children whom they leave under the temporary care of the facility (chapter 5).

25. The facility shall require that parents and guardians provide the facility with names of persons who are authorized by the parent or legal guardian to pick up each child. The facility shall not release children to any unauthorized person, and furthermore, the facility shall maintain records of the date and time each child checked out and was dropped off and the name of the person to whom the child was released (chapter 5).

26. Facilities shall have written policies regarding children's issues, such as requirements for staff providing supervision of children, age limits for children, restroom practices, food, and parental presence on site. Facilities shall inform parents and guardians of these policies and require that parents and guardians sign a form that acknowledges that they have received the policies, understand the policies, and will abide by the policies (chapter 5).

(continued)

27. Facilities, to the extent required by law, must adhere to the standards of building design that relate to the designing, building, expanding, or renovating of space as detailed in the Americans with Disabilities Act (ADA) (chapter 6).

28. Facilities must be in compliance with all federal, state, and local building codes (chapter 6).

29. The aquatic and pool facilities must provide the proper safety equipment according to state and local codes and regulations (chapter 7).

30. Facility operators shall post proper caution, danger, and warning signage in conspicuous locations where facility staff know, or should know, that existing conditions and situations warrant such signage (chapter 8).

31. Facility operators shall post the appropriate emergency and safety signage pertaining to fire and related emergency situations, as required by federal, state, and local codes (chapter 8).

32. Facility operators shall post signage indicating the location of any AED and first-aid kits, including directions on how to access those locations (chapter 8).

33. Facilities shall post all ADA and OSHA signage that is required by federal, state, and local laws and regulations (chapter 8).

34. All cautionary, danger, and warning signage shall have the required signal icon, signal word, signal color, and layout as specified in ASTM F1749 (chapter 8).

TABLE A.2   Guidelines for Health/Fitness Facilities

1. Prospective members and/or users who fail to complete the pre-activity screening procedures on request should be permitted to sign a waiver or release that allows them to participate in the program offerings of the facility. In those instances where such members and/or users refuse to sign a release or waiver, they should be excluded from participation to the extent permitted by law (chapter 1).

2. All members or users who have been identified (either through a pre-activity screening or by self-disclosure to a qualified healthcare and/or health/fitness professional on staff) as having cardiovascular, metabolic, or pulmonary disease or symptoms or any other potentially serious medical concern (e.g., orthopedic problems) and who subsequently fail to get consultation should be permitted to sign a waiver or release that allows them to participate in the facility's program offerings. In those situations where such members or users refuse to sign a waiver or release, they should be excluded from participation to the extent permitted by law (chapter 1).

3. Facilities should provide new and existing members with the opportunity to receive personal instruction and guidance with regard to their physical activity programs (chapter 2).

4. Facilities should provide members with ongoing monitoring of their physical activity programs, including the opportunity to receive guidance on adjusting their physical activity programs (chapter 2).

5. Depending on their targeted audiences, facility operators should consider providing an array of physical activity options to accommodate the physical, emotional, and personal preferences of each user of the facility (chapter 2).

6. Staffed facilities should provide professional health/fitness staff to supervise the fitness floor during peak usage periods (chapter 2).

7. Facilities should use waivers of liability and/or assumption of risk documents with all facility members and users (chapter 3).

8. A facility that delivers or prescribes physical activity programs, primarily or exclusively, to members and users who are considered at an elevated risk for experiencing a health-related event because of their participation in physical activity (e.g., users over the age of 50, individuals with coronary risk factors, diabetes, or clinical obesity) should have a medical director, a medical liaison, or a medical advisory committee provide assistance in reviewing the facility's physical activity screening and programming protocols as well its emergency response protocols (chapter 3).

9. Facilities should provide the appropriate level of supervision and monitoring for each of the physical activity areas in the facility (chapter 3).

10. All physical activity areas should have a clock, a chart of target heart rates, and a chart depicting ratings of perceived exertion to enable members and users to monitor their level of physical exertion (chapter 3).

11. A facility should extend to each employee on staff the opportunity to receive training and certification in first aid and the use of CPR and an AED (chapter 3).

12. Facilities should have an incident report system that provides written documentation of all incidents that occur within the facility or within the facility's scope of responsibility. Such reports should be completed in a timely fashion and maintained on file, according to the regulatory statute of limitations for the location in which the facility does business (chapter 3).

13. Facility operators should consider having health/fitness professionals who have the appropriate level of professional education and/or certification to assess and prescribe physical activity for individuals with special needs (chapter 4).

14. Facility operators should consider having all staff members trained and certified in cardiopulmonary resuscitation and AED administration (chapter 4).

15. Facility operators should perform criminal background checks on employees and independent contractors who have responsibilities that involve working with youth or whose responsibilities involve personal contact with members and users or other employees in an unsupervised environment (chapter 4).

16. Facilities that are staffed during all operating hours should have a manager on duty (MOD) or supervisor on duty (SOD) schedule that specifies which professional staff person has supervisory responsibility overseeing all operating activities during the hours that the facility is open (chapter 5).

17. Facility operators who operate under a staffed business model should provide the proper level of qualified staffing in nonactivity areas to assist in serving the members and users and providing support to emergency response situations that might arise (chapter 5).

18. Facilities that are unstaffed during some or all operating hours, and therefore have periods in which no supervision is offered, should provide the appropriate signage to communicate to members and users that the facility is unsupervised, the inherent risks in using the facility, and what steps the members and users should take in the event of a witnessed emergency situation (chapter 5).

19. Facilities should have a written system for cleaning and disinfecting the various areas in the facility (chapter 5).

20. Designers should size both physical activity spaces and non-activity spaces to provide sufficient space to accommodate the expected user demand (chapter 6).

21. Designers should configure physical activity space plans so that defined circulation routes are adjacent to, rather than through, the various activity zones (chapter 6).

22. Facilities should provide open-access circulation, which avoids blind corners, unnecessary doors, partitions, and other hazards that would present a safety risk to members and users (chapter 6).

23. Designers should separate physical activity spaces from operational, storage, and maintenance spaces (chapter 6).

24. Facilities should provide all physical activity spaces with sufficient air circulation and fresh makeup air (i.e., outside air) to maintain air quality, room temperatures, and humidity at safe and comfortable levels. Notable exceptions to this particular guideline include such spaces as saunas, steam rooms, and hot yoga studios. However, even in these particular areas, measures to ensure safe and healthy human occupancy must be understood and implemented (chapter 6).

25. Facilities should illuminate all facility spaces to allow members and users to safely engage in their physical activity regimens. Minimum safe illumination levels vary according to activity in a particular area and should be carefully researched. The emerging need for energy conservation requires lighting solutions that take advantage of the available daylighting sources, automatic control devices, and the latest technologies in lamp and fixture design (chapter 6).

(continued)

26. Facilities should be designed to maintain background noise levels below 70 decibels and never above 90 decibels. Sound transmission through defining perimeter partitions of a noise-generating activity area should be limited to a level that does not adversely affect the functionality level of neighboring spaces (chapter 6).

27. Floor surfaces in physical activity areas should meet specifications regarding the proper level of absorption and slip resistance to minimize the risk of fall-related injuries (chapter 6).

28. Facilities should have wall surfaces in activity spaces that are nonabrasive, flush, and free of protrusions that could cause impact injuries. Activity spaces that involve airborne projectiles, such as volleyballs or basketballs, should have a perimeter ball-containment barrier to protect users in adjacent areas and walkways (chapter 6).

29. When physical activity spaces have depth and distance parameters that can affect an individual's safety, then the facility should provide appropriate markings to ensure that users are aware of these depth and distance parameters (chapter 6).

30. Facilities should use "green" design and sustainable construction materials and techniques. Regardless of whether official certification is a desired goal, the widely published principles of green design related to site development, storm-water management, energy conservation, renewable resources, water conservation, indoor air quality, carbon reduction, and pollution control should be honored, whenever possible (chapter 6).

31. Facility operators should provide a sufficient quantity and quality of equipment so that the facility is able to fulfill its mission, purpose, and intended function for its targeted members and users (chapter 7).

32. Facility operators should have a preventive maintenance program for their fitness equipment, including documentation showing when the scheduled work was performed (chapter 7).

33. Facility operators should have a system in place for removing broken or damaged equipment from member use until that equipment has been repaired or replaced (chapter 7).

34. All physical activity areas should have a clock, a chart of target heart rates, and a chart depicting ratings of perceived exertion to enable members and users to monitor their level of physical exertion (chapter 7).

35. Facility operators should consider providing a few pieces of fitness equipment that can be accessed by individuals with physical limitations who require the use of a wheelchair, including at least one piece of cardiovascular equipment and one piece of selectorized or variable-resistance equipment (chapter 7).

36. Facilities should provide message boards, bulletin boards, electronic bulletin boards, websites, or a similar type of communication venue for the communication and dissemination of relevant information on the facility or of particular interest to the facility's members (chapter 8).

37. Signage should have the proper appearance, readability, and placement in order to clearly display the desired message in a fashion that can easily be understood by the intended audience (chapter 8).

APPENDIX B

Supplements

Supplement 1

Lighting Guidelines for Selected Outdoor Areas and Activities

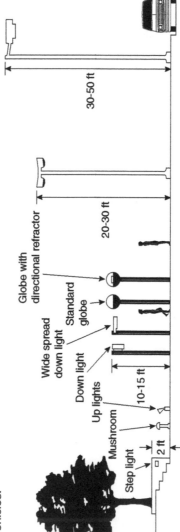

Considerations

The following factors must be considered when installing or renovating outdoor lighting systems:

1. In general, overhead lighting is more efficient and economical than low-level lighting.

2. Fixtures should provide an overlapping pattern of light at a height of about 7 ft.

3. Lighting levels should respond to site hazards such as steps, ramps, and steep embankments.

4. Posts and standards should be placed so that they do not create hazards for pedestrians or vehicles.

Notes

1. Because of their effect on light distribution, trees and shrubs at present height and growth potential should be considered in a lighting layout.

2. It is recommended that facilities use manufacturer-provided lighting templates sized for fixture type, wattage, pole height, and layout scale.

3. Facilities should consider color rendition when selecting light source. When possible, colors should be selected under proposed light source.

4. Light pollution to areas other than those to be illuminated should be avoided.

Low-level lighting

1. Heights below eye level

2. Very finite patterns with low wattage capabilities

3. Incandescent, fluorescent, and high-pressure sodium, 5- to 150-W lamps

4. Lowest maintenance requirements, but highly susceptible to vandals

Mall and walkway lighting

1. 10- to 15-ft heights average for multiuse areas; wide variety of fixtures and light patterns

2. Mercury, metal halide, or high-pressure sodium, 70- to 250-W lamps

3. Susceptible to vandals

Special-purpose lighting

1. 20- to 30-ft heights average

2. Recreational, commercial, residential, and industrial

3. Mercury, metal halide, or high-pressure sodium, 200- to 400-W lamps

4. Fixtures maintained by gantry

Parkway and roadway lighting

1. 30- to 50-ft heights average

2. Large recreational, commercial, and industrial areas, and highways

3. Mercury, metal halide, or high-pressure sodium, 400- to 1000-W lamps

4. Fixtures maintained by gantry

High mastlighting

1. 60- to 100-ft heights average

2. Large areas—parking and recreational areas and highway interchanges

3. Metal halide or high-pressure sodium, 1000-W lamps

4. Fixtures must lower for maintenance

Globe with directional refractor
Wide spread down light
Standard globe
Down light
Up lights
Mushroom
Step light
2 ft
10-15 ft
20-30 ft
30-50 ft
60-100 ft

Architectural graphic standards, 8th ed., C.G. Ramsey and H.R. Sleeper. Copyright 1988 by John Wiley & Sons, Inc. Reprinted by permission of John Wiley & Sons, Inc.

Samples of Signage Used in a Health/Fitness Facility

Sauna Policies

1. The sauna temperature is kept between 170 and 180 °F (77 and 82 °C).
2. Limit yourself to a maximum of 10 minutes.
3. Because of high temperatures, the sauna can be dangerous to your health. We recommend that you consult your physician before you use the sauna. Those who are pregnant and those with medical conditions such as high blood pressure, heart disease, and respiratory problems should avoid exposure to high heat.
4. Allow yourself at least 5 minutes after exercising to cool down before entering.
5. No food or drink is allowed inside.
6. Please shower before entering.

Steam Room Policies

1. The steam room temperature is kept between 100 and 110 °F (38 and 43 °C).
2. Limit yourself to a maximum of 10 minutes.
3. Because of high temperatures and humidity, the steam room can be dangerous to your health. We recommend that you consult your physician before you use the steam room. Those who are pregnant and those with medical conditions such as high blood pressure, heart disease, and respiratory problems should avoid exposure to high heat and humidity.
4. Allow yourself at least 5 minutes after exercising to cool down before entering.
5. No food or drink is allowed inside.
6. Please shower before entering.

Pool Policies

1. The pool temperature is kept between 78 and 84 °F (25 and 29 °C) and is posted daily.
2. Please shower before entering the pool.
3. No diving is allowed.
4. No food or drink is allowed in the pool area.
5. No running or playing is allowed on the pool deck.
6. Individuals with open wounds or sores should not enter the pool.

Racquetball Court Rules

1. Eye guards are required!
2. Black-soled shoes are not allowed on the court.
3. No food or drink is allowed on the court.

Court Numbers Signs

Racquetball Court 1   Squash Court 1
Racquetball Court 2   Squash Court 2
Racquetball Court 3   Squash Court 3

Cardiovascular Area Policies

1. Please limit yourself to 30 minutes on all cardiovascular equipment. During prime times, limit yourself to 20 minutes.
2. Please use the sign-up board when all equipment is taken so people can use the equipment on a first-come, first-served basis.
3. Please wipe off controls, seats, and railings when you are finished with your workout.
4. Please return cardiovascular equipment controls to their start position when your workout is completed.
5. We recommend you see the club's fitness staff before you start a training program.
6. Please warm up before using the equipment and cool down afterward.
7. Please report any injuries to the facility staff.

Resistance Circuit Policies

1. We recommend you see the club's fitness staff before you start a training program.
2. During prime times, please limit yourself to a maximum of two sets per station. You may return after completing the rest of your circuit.
3. Please lower and raise the plates carefully.
4. Please wipe off the pads when you are finished with a piece of equipment.

Free Weight Area Policies

1. We recommend you see the club's fitness staff before you start a training program.
2. Because of the high risk of injury, we recommend you use a spotter when training with free weights.

(continued)

(continued)

3. Please replace all dumbbells and plates on the appropriate racks when finished with them.

4. Please remove plates from bars when you are finished with them.

Treadmill Policies

1. Start the treadmill before you step on the belt.

2. Increase the speed and elevation gradually.

3. After completing your workout, gradually reduce the speed to 3 miles per hour and the elevation to 0.

4. Please wipe off the control panel after completing your workout.

Pool Temperature

1. Pool temperature is _____.

(The blank should be filled in with signage of temperature. Facility operators should create temperature figures from 78 to 86 °F.)

Whirlpool Policies

1. The whirlpool temperature is kept between 102 and 105 °F.

2. Limit yourself to a maximum of 10 minutes.

3. Due to high temperature and humidity, the whirlpool can be dangerous to your health. We recommend that you consult your physician before you use the whirlpool. Those who are pregnant and those with medical conditions such as high blood pressure, heart disease, and respiratory problems should avoid exposure to high heat and humidity.

4. Allow yourself at least 5 minutes after exercising to cool down before entering.

5. No food or drink is allowed in whirlpool.

6. Please shower before entering.

Equipment Out of Order

This equipment is out of service. It will be repaired or in service by _____.

Supplement 3

Sample Preventive Maintenance Schedule— Resistance Equipment

Equipment	Daily	Weekly	Monthly
Selectorized	Clean upholstery with cotton cloth and mild soap solution. Clean frames with cotton cloth and either warm mild detergent or all-purpose liquid cleaner. *Extra* Clean off dumbbell rack with warm mild detergent or all-purpose liquid cleaner.	Lubricate guide rods and linear bearings (wipe clean with dry cotton cloth, then wipe entire length with medium weight oil). Inspect and adjust the following: • Cables • Nuts and bolts • Torn upholstery Apply vinyl upholstery protectant. *Extra* Wipe off dumbbells and barbell plates. Check bolts on bars.	Wash grips in mild soap and water.
Pneumatic	Clean upholstery with cotton cloth and mild soap solution. Wipe off frames with cotton cloth. Release air pressure.	Polish chrome with cotton cloth and automotive chrome polish. Clean seat belts with mild soap. Every two weeks, switch the compressor pump. Apply vinyl upholstery protectant.	Lubricate cylinder rods with dry cotton cloth and lightweight machine oil. Lubricate pivot bearings. Wash rubber handgrips in mild soap and water.

Supplement 4

Sample Preventive Maintenance Schedule—Cardiovascular Equipment

Equipment	Daily	Weekly	Monthly	Biannually
Rower	Clean monorail with nonabrasive pad. Wipe off seat and console with 100% cotton cloth using water and mild detergent (dilute).	Clean and lubricate chain using 100% cotton cloth and lightweight oil. Clean pads with vinyl protectant.	Inspect chain links. Adjust seat rollers. Inspect chain handle. Tighten shock cord.	Replace monitor batteries.
Arm/leg ergometer	Wipe off seat and console with 100% cotton cloth plus water and mild detergent. Rinse.	Clean and lubricate chain with cotton cloth and lightweight machine oil. Clean seat with vinyl protectant.	Inspect bolts.	
Computerized bike	Clean seat and console with 100% cotton cloth and mild soap with water (dilute). Clean housing with same materials.	Clean and lubricate chain with cotton cloth and lightweight machine oil. Clean pedals and lubricate. Wax seat post with auto wax. Clean shroud and seat with vinyl protectant.	Inspect bolts and screws.	
Mechanical stairclimber	Clean console and housing with cotton cloth and water with mild detergent. Wipe and clean pedals and grips with same solution.	Clean and lubricate all bushings with lightweight machine oil. Clean machine with vinyl protectant.	Inspect housing, belts, and electrical components and repair as needed.	
Treadmill	Clean console and housing with cotton cloth and water with mild detergent solution.	Clean belt with cotton cloth and mild detergent solution. Must run belt at 2 mph while cleaning.	Inspect electrical components and bolts—calibrate if needed (see manual).	
Recumbent bike	Clean housing, console, and seat with cotton cloth and mild soap. Charge battery overnight.	Inspect all bolts and chains and adjust as needed.		

Outline for a Hazard Communication Program

The OSHA Hazard Communication Standard requires you to develop a written hazard communication program. The following is an outline of how to set up your hazard communication.

1. **General company policy.** This must state the organization's intent to comply with OSHA Hazard Communication Standard, Title 29, Code of Federal Regulations 1920.1200. This section should provide an overview of the organization's policy.

2. **List of hazardous chemicals.** This must list chemicals and their locations. It should also mention that lists of chemicals will be posted in the appropriate facility areas.

3. **Material safety data sheets.** This must outline what the chemical compositions and safety hazards of a product are, how they will be posted, and who is in charge.

4. **Labels and other forms of warning.** This section must clearly state that labels and other warnings will be posted on all hazardous materials.

5. **Nonroutine tasks.** This section must describe precautions and training that will be required for nonroutine tasks.

6. **Training.** This section must outline the organization's initial and ongoing training programs that pertain to use and handling of hazardous materials.

7. **Contractor employees.** This section must outline policies for dealing with independent contractors.

8. **Additional information.** This section must direct employees to the appropriate information source for further data.

Supplement 6

Acoustical Guidelines for a Health/Fitness Facility

Owners and managers of health/fitness facilities should incorporate the following noise guidelines into the design and operation of the health/fitness facility.

Area	STC rating	Measured reverberation time
Aerobic studio	45 to 55	0.8 to 1.4 s
Control desk	45 to 50	0.8 to 1.4 s
Cardiovascular training area	40 to 50	0.8 to 1.4 s
Resistance training area	40 to 50	0.8 to 1.4 s
Free-weight area	40 to 50	0.8 to 1.4 s
Gymnasium	45 to 55	0.8 to 1.4 s
Racquetball court	45 to 55	0.8 to 1.4 s
Squash court	45 to 55	0.8 to 1.4 s
Indoor pool	45 to 55	0.8 to 1.4 s
Locker rooms	45 to 50	0.8 to 1.4 s
Pro shop area	60 minimum	0.8 to 1.4 s
Massage	45 to 55	0.8 to 1.4 s
Sports/physical therapy	45 to 55	0.8 to 1.4 s
Playroom	50 to 55	0.8 to 1.4 s
Offices	50 to 55	0.8 to 1.4 s
Storage	40 to 45	0.8 to 1.4 s
Indoor tennis courts	45 to 55	0.8 to 1.4 s
Laundry area	50 to 60	0.8 to 1.4 s
Indoor track area	45 to 55	0.8 to 1.4 s

RATIONALE
SOUND CONTROL OBJECTIVES

The primary reasons for attempting to control noise within the health/fitness facility involve either increasing the comfort level for facility employees and users or improving communications between occupants of the facility. Although little to no threat of hearing loss from sound abuses exists within the health/fitness facility, high noise levels do cause other problems. Noise can be disruptive and is usually irritating. Noise also hinders an individual's sense of privacy. Perhaps most important, noise can have a negative effect on task performance.

NOISE STANDARDS

Noise is generally measured with sound-pressure meters that record sound in decibels (dB). Minimal acceptable standards for safe noise levels have been established by two federal regulatory agencies—the Occupational Safety and Health Administration (OSHA) and the Environmental Protection Agency (EPA).

NOISE SOLUTIONS

Excessive noise levels can be reduced to acceptable levels by specific actions depending upon the cause of the noise. The two primary sources of unwanted sound—high noise levels and excessive reverberation—can be dampened by adding acoustical absorbents in the affected areas. The degree of insulation of airborne sound provided by a given material is indicated by its sound transmission class (STC) rating. The higher the rating, the better the level of sound absorption. Other methods for diminishing unwanted sound include changing the shape or the layout of an area, using background sound to mask the noise, directly eliminating the cause of the noise (e.g., the stereo system may be too loud), and isolating either the sound or the vibration.

Recommended Maximum Background Noise Criterion Curves for Health and Fitness Facilities

Facility area	NC level	Facility area	NC level
Exercise classroom	35-40	Child care	25-35
Fitness floor	35-40	Racket courts	35-40
Gymnasium	35-40	Pools (indoor)	35-40
Locker rooms	35-40	Offices	30-35
Physical therapy	30-35		

Note: The noise criteria (NC) curves provide a convenient way of defining ambient noise level in terms of octave band sound pressure levels. The NC curves consist of a family of curves relating the spectrum of noise to an environment. Therefore, higher noise levels (decibels) may be allowed at lower frequencies because the ear is less sensitive to noise at lower frequencies.

Architectural graphic standards, 8th ed., C.G. Ramsey and H.R. Sleeper. Copyright 1988 by John Wiley & Sons, Inc. Reprinted by permission of John Wiley & Sons, Inc.

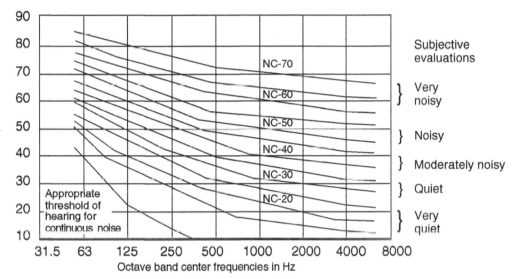

Architectural graphic standards, 8th ed., C.G. Ramsey and H.R. Sleeper. Copyright 1988 by John Wiley & Sons, Inc. Reprinted by permission of John Wiley & Sons, Inc.

Noise Criteria Sound Pressure Level Table

	SOUND PRESSURE LEVEL, DB							
NC curve	63 Hz	125 Hz	250 Hz	500 Hz	1000 Hz	2000 Hz	4000 Hz	8000 Hz
NC-70	83	79	75	72	71	70	69	68
NC-65	80	75	71	68	66	64	63	62
NC-60	77	71	67	63	61	59	58	57
NC-55	74	67	62	58	56	54	53	52
NC-50	71	64	58	54	51	49	48	47
NC-45	67	60	54	49	46	44	43	42
NC-40	64	57	50	45	41	39	38	37
NC-35	60	52	45	40	36	34	33	32
NC-30	57	48	41	36	31	29	28	27
NC-25	54	44	37	31	27	24	22	21
NC-20	50	41	33	26	22	19	17	16
NC-15	47	36	29	22	17	14	12	11

Note: For convenience in using noise criteria data, the table lists the sound pressure levels in decibels for the NC curves from the above chart.

Architectural graphic standards, 8th ed., C.G. Ramsey and H.R. Sleeper. Copyright 1988 by John Wiley & Sons, Inc. Reprinted by permission of John Wiley & Sons, Inc.

Supplement 7

Effects of Various Temperatures on Human Performance

Effective temperature (F°)*	Performance effects
90	Upper limit for continued occupancy over any reasonable period of time.
80-90	Expect universal complaints, serious mental and psychomotor performance decrement, and physical fatigue.
80	Maximum for acceptable performance even of limited work; work output reduced as much as 40 to 50%; most people experience nasal dryness.
78	Regular decrement in psychomotor performance; individuals experience difficulty falling asleep and remaining asleep; optimum for bathing or showering.
75	Clothed subjects experience physical fatigue, become lethargic and sleepy, and feel warm; unclothed subjects consider this temperature optimum without some type of protective cover.
72	Preferred for year-round sedentary activity while subjects are wearing light clothing.
70	Midpoint for summer comfort; optimum for demanding visual-motor tasks.
68	Midpoint for winter comfort (heavier clothing) and moderate activity, but slight deterioration in kinesthetic response; people begin to feel cool indoors while performing sedentary activities.
66	Midpoint for winter comfort (very heavy clothing) while subjects are performing heavy work or vigorous physical exercise.
64	Lower limit for acceptable motor coordination; shivering occurs if individuals are not extremely active.
60	Hand and finger dexterity deteriorates, limb stiffness begins to occur, and shivering is positive.
55	Hand dexterity is reduced by 50%, strength is materially decreased, and there is considerable (probably uncontrolled) shivering.
50	Extreme stiffness; strength application accompanied by some pain; lower limit for unprotected exposure for more than a few minutes.

*These temperature effects are based on relatively still air and normal humidity (40 to 60%). Higher temperatures are acceptable if airflow is increased and humidity is lowered (a shift from 1 to 4°); lower temperatures are less acceptable if airflow increases (a shift upward of 1 to 2°).

Supplement 8
General Illumination Guidelines

Task requirements	Light level (FC)	Type of illumination
Small detail; low contrast; prolonged viewing; fast, error-free response	100	Supplementary lighting fixture located near visual task
Small detail, fair contrast, close but short duration work, speed not essential	50-100	Supplementary lighting and/or well-distributed and diffused general lighting
Typical office/desk activity	40-60	General lighting with diffusing fixture directly overhead
Sports (e.g., tennis and basketball) or indoor recreational games (e.g., Ping-Pong and billiards)	30-50	General lighting with sufficient number of fixtures to provide even court or table illumination
Recreational reading and letter writing	25-45	Supplementary lighting, positioned over reading so that page glare does not occur
Typical housekeeping activities	10-25	General lighting
Visibility for moving about, avoiding people and furniture, and negotiating standard stairs	5-10	General and/or supplementary lighting (with care taken not to allow supplementary sources to project in the user's eyes)

Note: These guidelines are only approximations. Foot-candle values are higher than some recommendations, not for seeing, but because these levels provide an additional psychological benefit as well. Levels relate to light levels measured at the primary seeing point (e.g., the desk or table surface, on the floor, or stair tread level). Brightness ratios between the seeing task and the immediate surroundings should not exceed 5:1; between the task and the remote surroundings, 20:1; and between the immediate work area and any other remaining visual environment, 80:1. Natural or white artificial light should be used regardless of the type of illumination (i.e., these levels do not apply to monochromatic light sources).

Supplement 9

DIN Floor Standards

The flooring for a multiuse exercise area should adhere to Deutsches Institut für Normung (DIN) standards. These standards require that a floor meet six criteria:

1. **Shock absorption**—a floor's ability to reduce the impact of contact with the floor surface. The greater the shock absorption, the more protective it is because it reduces impact forces. An aerobics floor, for example, would need more shock absorption than a basketball court.

2. **Standard vertical deformation**—the actual vertical deflection of the floor upon impact. The greater the deformation, the more the floor defects downward. Floors with minimal deformation are not good at absorbing impact forces.

3. **Deflective indentation**—the actual vertical deflection of the floor at a distance 50 cm from the point of impact. The greater the indentation, the more likely impact at one spot will cause deflection at a distant point.

4. **Sliding characteristics**—the surface friction of the finished floor. A floor with poor sliding characteristics would be inappropriate for aerobics or basketball.

5. **Ball reflection (game-action response)**—the response of a ball dropped on the floor compared to a ball dropped on concrete.

6. **Rolling load**—a floor's ability to withstand heavy weight without breaking or sustaining permanent damage.

These DIN criteria are then used to evaluate the effectiveness of a floor. A floor will have one of three functions:

1. **Sports function**—A floor that serves a sports function enhances athletic performance. Surface friction and ball reflection are important here.

2. **Protective function**—A floor that serves a protective function reduces the risk of injury (e.g., from a fall) during activity. Shock absorption is important here.

3. **Material–technical function**—A floor that serves a material–technical function meets the sports and protective functions.

In a health/fitness facility, the gymnasium and multipurpose floors are classified under sports function or material–technical function. The aerobics floor is classified under protective function, with some sports function characteristics.

A floor surface that has a material–technical function should meet the following DIN criteria:

Shock absorption	53% minimum
Standard vertical deformation	2.3 mm minimum
Deflective indentation	15% maximum
Sliding characteristics	0.5 to 0.7 range
Ball deflection	90% minimum
Rolling load	337.6 lb (153.1 kg)

Supplement 10

Dimensions and Markings for a Basketball Court

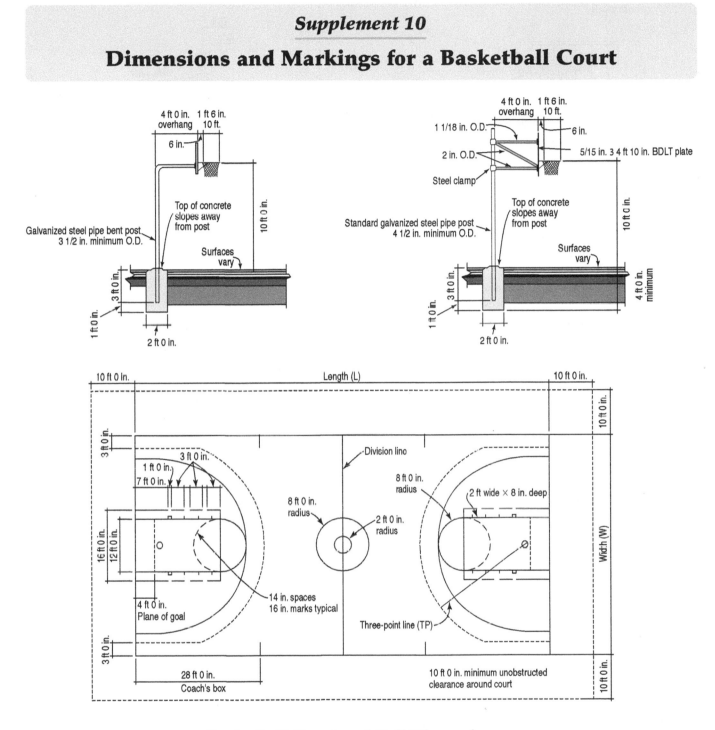

Basketball Court and Ball Dimensions

COURT				BASKETBALL		
Type	L (ft)	W (ft)	TP (ft-In)	Type	Max circumference (in.)	Min. circumference (in.)
NBA	94	50	23-9 R	NBA	30	29.5
International	94	50	20-61 R	International	30	29.5
NCAA (men)	94	50	19-9 R	NCAA (men)	30	29.5
WNBA NCAA (women)	94	50	19-9 R	WNBA NCAA (women)	29	28.5
High school (men)	84	50	19-9 R	High school (men)	30	29.5
High school (women)	84	50	19-9 R	High school (women)	29	28.5

L = length, W = width, TP = three point line.

(continued)

(continued)

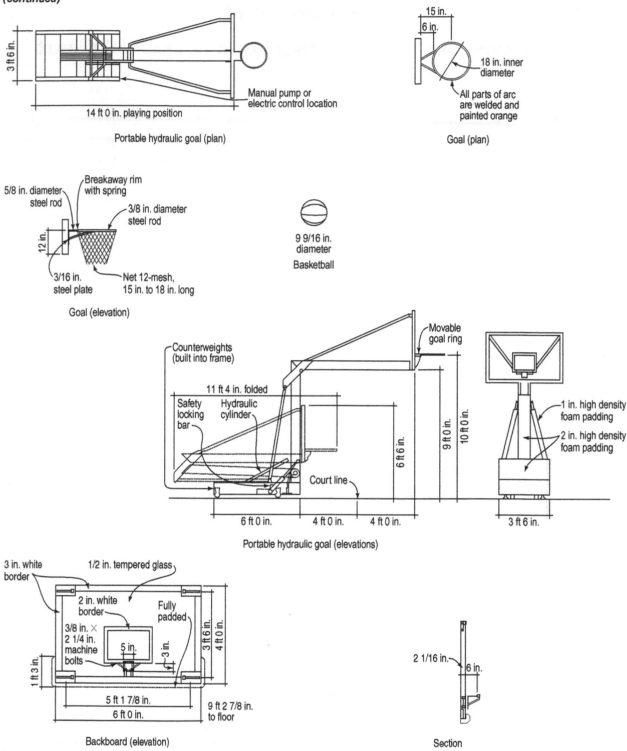

Portable hydraulic goal (plan)

Goal (plan)

15 in.

6 in.

18 in. inner diameter

All parts of arc are welded and painted orange

3 ft 6 in.

14 ft 0 in. playing position

Manual pump or electric control location

5/8 in. diameter steel rod

Breakaway rim with spring

3/8 in. diameter steel rod

12 in.

3/16 in. steel plate

Net 12-mesh, 15 in. to 18 in. long

Goal (elevation)

9 9/16 in. diameter

Basketball

Movable goal ring

Counterweights (built into frame)

11 ft 4 in. folded

Safety locking bar

Hydraulic cylinder

6 ft 6 in.

9 ft 0 in.

10 ft 0 in.

1 in. high density foam padding

2 in. high density foam padding

Court line

6 ft 0 in.

4 ft 0 in.

4 ft 0 in.

3 ft 6 in.

Portable hydraulic goal (elevations)

3 in. white border

1/2 in. tempered glass

2 in. white border

Fully padded

3/8 in. × 2 1/4 in. machine bolts

5 in.

3 in.

3 ft 6 in.

4 ft 0 in.

1 ft 3 in.

5 ft 1 7/8 in.

6 ft 0 in.

9 ft 2 7/8 in. to floor

Backboard (elevation)

2 1/16 in.

6 in.

Section

Note: A basketball court used in high school competition is generally 84 × 50 ft with a 10-ft unobstructed space on all sides (3-ft minimum). A basketball court used in colleges should be 94 ft × 50 ft, with a 10-ft unobstructed space on all sides (3-ft minimum). The color of the lane space marks and neutral zone marks should contrast with the color of the bounding lines. The mid-court marks should be the same color as the bounding lines. All lines should be 2-in. wide (neutral zone excluded). All dimensions are to inside edge of lines except as noted. The backboard should be of any rigid weather-resistant material. The front surface should be flat and painted white unless it is transparent. If the backboard is transparent, it should be marked with a 3-in.-wide white line around the border and an 18-in. × 24-in. target area bounded with a 2-in.-wide white line (De Chiara and Callendar, 1990).

Supplement 11

Dimensions and Markings for a Volleyball Court

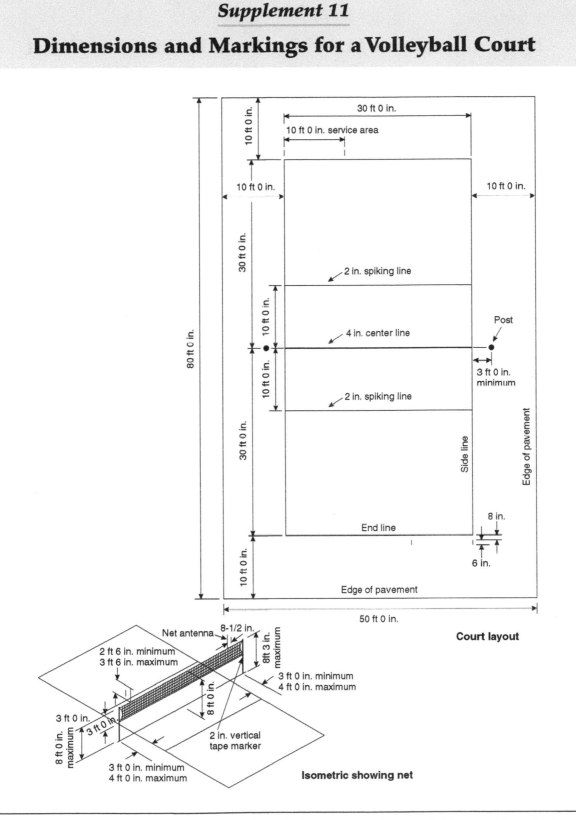

Court layout

Isometric showing net

Note: The recommended size of a volleyball court is 30 ft × 60 ft with a 10-ft unobstructed area on all sides (6 ft minimum). All measurements for court markings are to be outside of lines except for the centerline. All court markings are to be 2 in. wide, except as noted. Net height at center should be as follows: men 8 ft 0 in., women 7 ft 4 in., high school 7 ft 0 in., elementary school 6 ft 6 in.

Dimensions and Markings for a Badminton Court

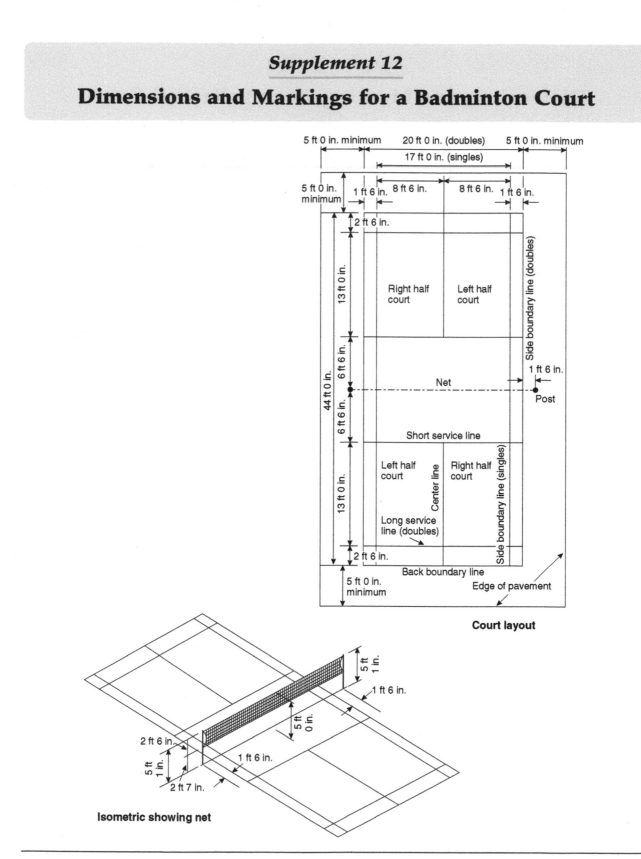

Court layout

Isometric showing net

Note: A singles court for badminton is 17 ft × 44 ft, whereas as doubles court is 20 ft × 44 ft. Both types of badminton courts should have a minimum unobstructed area of 5 ft on all sides. All measurements for court markings are to the outside of the lines except for those involving the center service line, which is equally divided between right and left service courts. All court markings should be 1 1/2 in. wide and preferably white or in color. Minimum distance between sides of parallel courts should be at least 5 ft.

Reprinted, by permission, from J. De Chiara and J.H. Callendar, 1990, *Time-saver standards for building types*, 3rd ed. (New York: McGraw-Hill Companies), 1192. © The McGraw-Hill Companies, Inc.

Supplement 13

Dimensions and Markings for a Racquetball and Handball Court

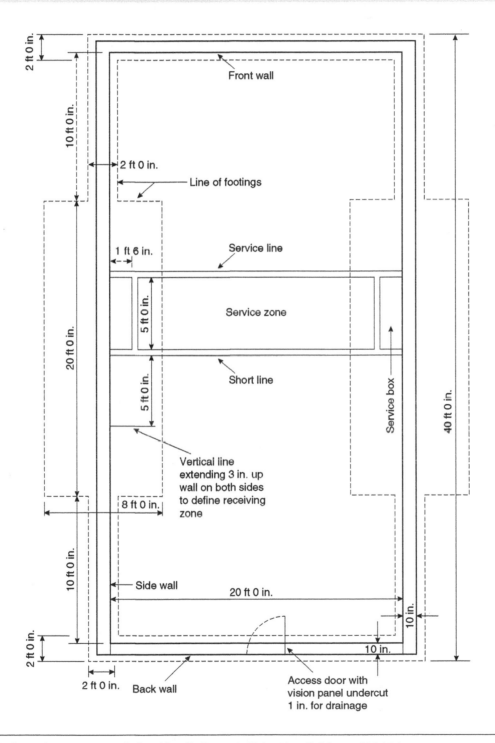

Front wall

2 ft 0 in.

10 ft 0 in.

2 ft 0 in.

Line of footings

1 ft 6 in.

Service line

5 ft 0 in.

Service zone

20 ft 0 in.

5 ft 0 in.

Short line

Service box

40 ft 0 in.

Vertical line extending 3 in. up wall on both sides to define receiving zone

8 ft 0 in.

10 ft 0 in.

Side wall

20 ft 0 in.

10 in.

2 ft 0 in.

2 ft 0 in.

Back wall

2 ft 0 in.

10 in.

Access door with vision panel undercut 1 in. for drainage

Note: A standard-size, four-wall racquetball and handball court is 20 ft wide × 40 ft long × 20 ft high. All court markings should be 1-1/2 in. wide and painted white, red, or yellow.

Reprinted, by permission, from J. De Chiara and J.H. Callendar, 1990, *Time-saver standards for building types*, 3rd ed. (New York: McGraw-Hill Companies), 1200. © The McGraw-Hill Companies, Inc.

Supplement 14

Dimensions and Markings for an International Singles and Doubles Squash Court

Singles squash court

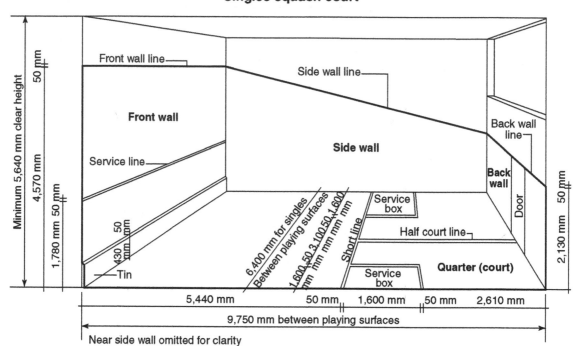

Near side wall omitted for clarity

Doubles squash court

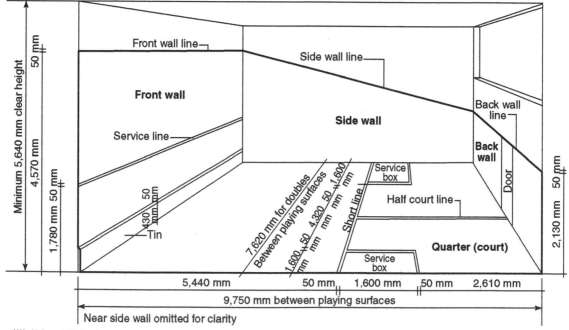

Near side wall omitted for clarity

Courtesy of World Squash Federation.

Dimensions for a Singles Squash Court

Length of court between playing surfaces	9,750 mm
Width of court between playing surfaces	6,400 mm
Diagonal	11,665 mm
Height above floor to lower edge of Front Wall Line	4,570 mm
Height above floor to lower edge of Back Wall Line	2,130 mm
Height above floor to lower edge of Service Line on Front Wall	1,780 mm
Height above floor to upper edge of the Tin	480 mm
Distance to nearest edge of Short Line from Back Wall	4,260 mm
Internal dimensions of Service Boxes	1,600 mm
Width of all lines and the upper section of the Tin	50 mm
Minimum clear height above the floor to the court	5,640 mm

Dimensions for a Doubles Squash Court

Length of court between playing surfaces	9,750 mm
Width of court between playing surfaces	7,620 mm or 8420 mm (Note 8)
Diagonal	12,375 mm
Height above floor to lower edge of Front Wall Line	4,570 mm
Height above floor to lower edge of Back Wall Line	2,130 mm
Height above floor to lower edge of Service Line on Front Wall	1,780 mm
Height above floor to upper edge of the Tin	480 mm
Distance to nearest edge of Short Line from Back Wall	4,260 mm
Internal dimensions of Service Boxes	1,600 mm
Width of all lines and the upper section of the Tin	50 mm
Minimum clear height above the floor to the court	5,640 mm

Notes

1. The Side Wall Line is angled between the Front Wall Line and the Back Wall Line.

2. The Service Box is a square formed by the Short Line, the Side Wall, and two other lines marked on the floor.

3. The length, width, and diagonal of the court are measured at a height of 1,000 mm above the floor.

4. It is recommended that the Front Wall Line, Side Wall Line, Back Wall Line, and upper 50 mm of the Tin are shaped so as to deflect any ball that strikes them.

5. No part of the upper section of the Tin shall project from the Front Wall by more than 45 mm.

6. It is recommended that the door to the court is in the center of the Back Wall.

7. The general configuration of a Squash Court, its dimensions, and its markings are illustrated on the diagrams on page 96.

8. For WSF recognized World and Regional events and Commonwealth Games, the width of the court between playing surfaces may be expanded from 7,620 mm to 8,420 mm.

Construction

A Squash Court may be constructed from a number of materials providing they have suitable ball rebound characteristics and are safe for play; however, the WSF publishes a Squash Court Specification, which contains recommended standards. The standards must be met for competitive play as required by the appropriate National Governing Body of Squash.

Court constructors are advised that where events involve professional players the height above floor to the top of the Tin may be reduced from 480mm to 430mm. If you are considering holding a professional tournament please check with the World Squash Federation office for the latest guidelines.

Supplement 15

Dimensions and Markings for a Tennis Court

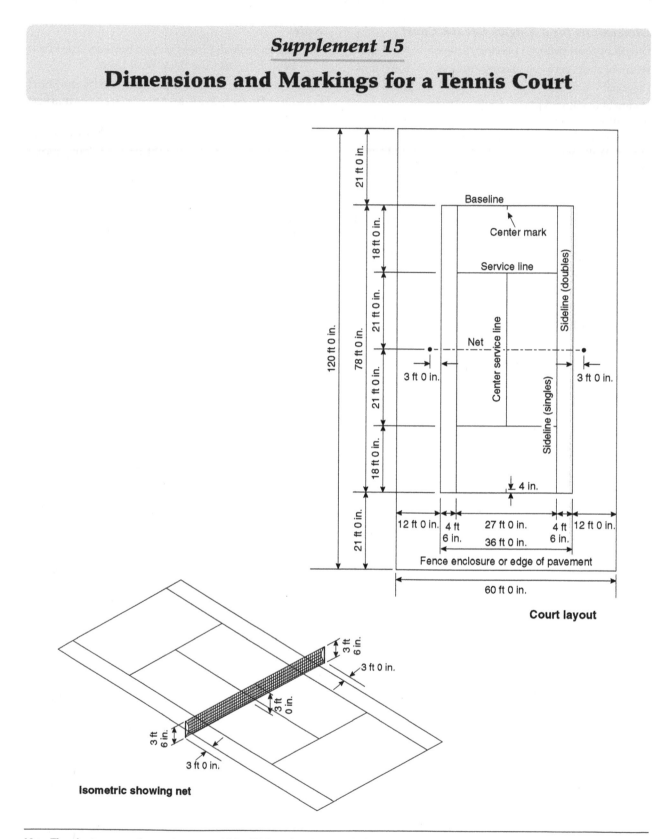

Court layout

Isometric showing net

Note: The playing area of a tennis court is 36 ft × 78 ft with at least 12 ft clearance on both sides or between a series of adjacent courts and 21 ft clearance on each end. All measurements for court markings are to the outside of lines except for those involving the center service line, which is equally divided between the right and left service courts. All court markings should be 2 in. wide. Fence enclosure, if provided, should be 10 ft high, 11-gauge, 1-3/4 in. mesh chain link.

Reprinted, by permission, from J. De Chiara and J.H. Callendar, 1990, *Time-saver standards for building types*, 3rd ed. (New York: McGraw-Hill Companies), 1210. © The McGraw-Hill Companies, Inc.

Supplement 16

Dimensions and Markings for a Platform Tennis Court

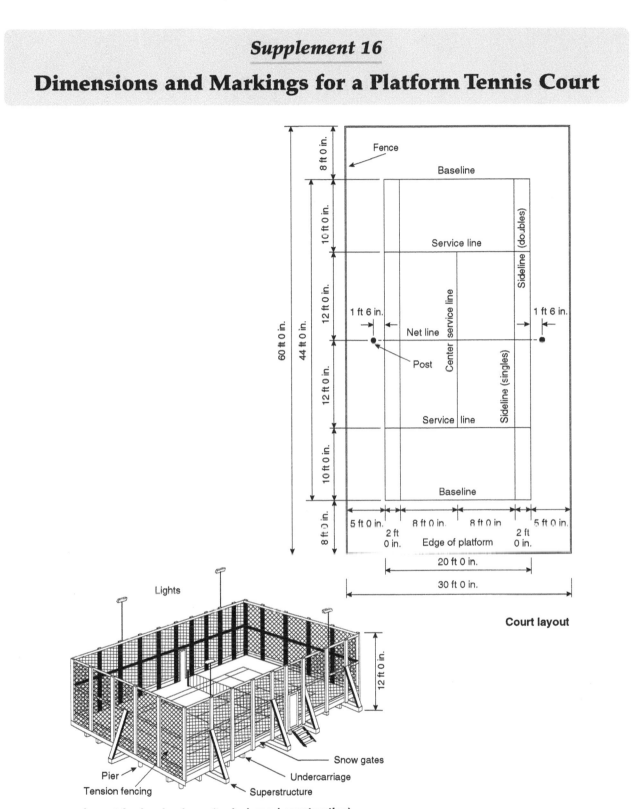

Court layout

Isometric showing fence (typical wood construction)

Note: The playing area of a platform tennis court is 20 ft × 44 ft, with an 8-ft space on each end and a 5-ft space on each side. All measurements for court markings are to be outside of lines except for those involving the center service line, which is equally divided between the right and left service court. All court markings should be 2 in. wide. Fencing is required—12 ft high with 16-gauge hexagonal, galvanized 1-in. flat wire mesh fabric. The net should be 3 ft 1 in. high at posts and 2 ft 10 in. at the center court.

Reprinted, by permission, from J. De Chiara and J.H. Callendar, 1990, *Time-saver standards for building types*, 3rd ed. (New York: McGraw-Hill Companies), 1208. © The McGraw-Hill Companies, Inc.

Supplement 17

Supplement 17

Dimensions and Markings for a Paddle Tennis Court

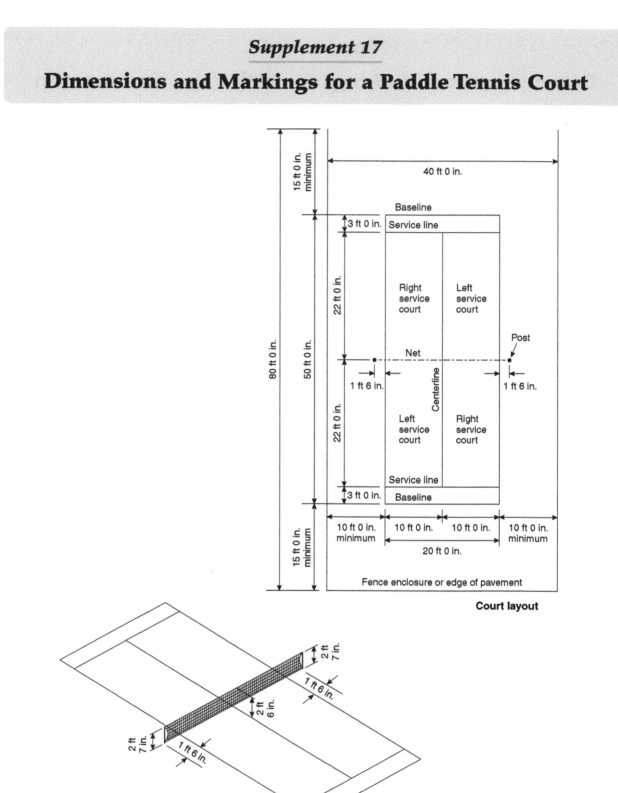

Court layout

Isometric showing net

Note: The playing area of a paddle tennis court is 20 ft × 50 ft, plus a 15-ft (minimum) space on each side and a 10-ft (minimum) space on each side or between an adjacent court. All measurements for court markings are to the outside of lines except for those involving the center service line, which is equally divided between the right and left service court. All court markings should be 1-1/2 in. wide. Fence enclosure, if provided, should be 1-1/2 in. mesh, 11-gauge chain link.

Reprinted, by permission, from J. De Chiara and J.H. Callendar, 1990, *Time-saver standards for building types*, 3rd ed. (New York: McGraw-Hill Companies), 1209. © The McGraw-Hill Companies, Inc.

Supplement 18

Illumination Requirements[1]
for Different Competitive Levels of Indoor Tennis Play

	ILLUMINATION LEVEL[2] FOR CLASS OF PLAY			
	I	II	III	IV
Description of the facility	Professional, international, national, and college	College, regional, municipal, club, and residential	Club, high school, instructional, parks, and residential	Parks and recreational
Average maintained horizontal illumination[3] within PPA (FC)	125	75	60	50
Minimum maintained horizontal illumination within PPA (FC)	100	60	50	40
Maximum uniformity ratio within primary playing area (FC) — CV	0.10 or less	0.10 or less	0.13 or less	0.17 or less
Maximum uniformity ratio within primary playing area (FC) — E_{max}/E_{min}	1.5:1 or less	1.5:1 or less	1.7:1 or less	2.0:1 or less

[1]Coordinated with the United States Tennis Association.

[2]Illuminance readings should be taken at a 1-meter (3-foot) elevation.

[3]Maintained minimum illuminance is the lowest maintained light level at any measurement or calculation point.

Material derived from the IESNA *Recommended Practice for Sports and Recreational Area Lighting*, with permission from IESNA.

Supplement 19

Illumination Requirements[1] for Different Competitive Levels of Outdoor Tennis Play

Description of the facility		ILLUMINATION LEVEL[2] FOR CLASS OF PLAY			
		I	II	III	IV
		Professional, international, national, and college	College, regional, municipal, club, and residential	Club, high school, instructional, parks, and residential	Parks and recreational
Average maintained horizontal illumination[3] within PPA (FC)		125	75	50	30
Minimum maintained horizontal illumination within PPA (FC)		100	60	40	20
Maximum uniformity ratio within primary playing area (FC)	CV	0.10 or less	0.13 or less	0.17 or less	0.21 or less
	E_{max}/E_{min}	1.5:1 or less	1.7:1 or less	2.1:1 or less	2.5:5 or less

[1]Coordinated with the United States Tennis Association.

[2]Illuminance readings should be taken at a 1-meter (3-foot) elevation.

[3]Maintained minimum illuminance is the lowest maintained light level at any measurement or calculation point.

Material derived from the IESNA *Recommended Practice for Sports and Recreational Area Lighting,* with permission from IESNA.

Supplement 20

Safety Checklist for Pool Areas

Inspection by _____ Date _____

Staff members are expected to report safety factors needing attention on a daily basis so that users are not exposed to unnecessary risks. Managers will make a complete written assessment of the condition of the facility on a regular basis.

Yes No

Lifesaving equipment

___ ___ Lifeguard stations are strategically located on decks near edge of pool.

___ ___ Shepherd's crooks, spine boards, reaching poles, and ring buoys are consistently placed in a conspicuous and appropriate location.

Pool and deck areas

___ ___ All deck areas are in safe condition.

___ ___ The decks are free of standing water.

___ ___ The sunbathing area is free of any dangerous conditions.

___ ___ The fence that encloses the pool area is in safe condition.

___ ___ All rules and regulations are posted in high-traffic areas such as entrances to the locker rooms. Special rules and regulations such as those on using the diving boards are posted in appropriate locations.

___ ___ All diving boards and stands are properly anchored and in good condition.

___ ___ Water clarity is such that the main drain is clearly visible on the bottom of the pool from the pool deck.

___ ___ All pool markings (depth/warning signs) are clearly visible.

___ ___ All matting on guard platforms is fastened securely and is in safe condition.

___ ___ Diving board steps and railings are fastened securely and are in safe condition.

___ ___ All chairs, cots, and lounges are in safe condition.

Guard room

___ ___ A copy of the procedures for emergencies is posted next to the telephone.

___ ___ Emergency phone numbers are also posted next to the telephone.

___ ___ A first-aid kit with all the necessary emergency first-aid essentials is consistently stored in a conspicuous location.

(continued)

(continued)

Filter and chlorinator rooms

___ ___ All motor shafts and filter and soda ash pumps are covered with metal guards.

___ ___ Fire extinguishers (Type B or C), filled and sealed and with current date tags, are kept in strategic locations.

___ ___ All chemicals are stored according to the manufacturer's storage instructions.

___ ___ Antichlorine gas mask is in operative condition. Mask is located immediately outside the entrance to the chlorine room. Canister element has a current, valid date.

___ ___ All gas chlorine tanks are fastened to the wall.

___ ___ Covers to powdered chemicals are fastened tightly and containers are neatly stored.

Locker rooms

___ ___ All floors are kept as dry as possible and are inspected for possible slippery or unsafe conditions.

___ ___ Basket/locker racks are secured to the wall or floor base and are in safe condition.

___ ___ Baskets are in place in the racks.

___ ___ All benches are secured to the wall. Bench tops are finished and free of any rough, splintered edges.

___ ___ All bather signs for pool users are displayed on the walls at appropriate heights.

___ ___ All shower-room plumbing is securely fastened to the walls, and is in safe and operable condition.

___ ___ All walls and ceilings are in safe condition.

___ ___ All lamps light when the switches are turned on.

Note: Completed checklists are valuable for several reasons. They are important tools for eliminating the avoidable injury. They also are tangible evidence that a pool manager has concern for the health and safety of pool patrons. In litigation alleging that an unsafe condition on the premises was the cause of the plaintiff's injuries, a completed checklist, signed and dated, could be invaluable. This checklist is incomplete. The items included are examples of safety checks that should be made. To be complete, the checklist should be tailored to a particular facility. Records of safety inspections should be kept indefinitely.

Supplement 21

Dimensions and Markings for a 25-Yard Pool

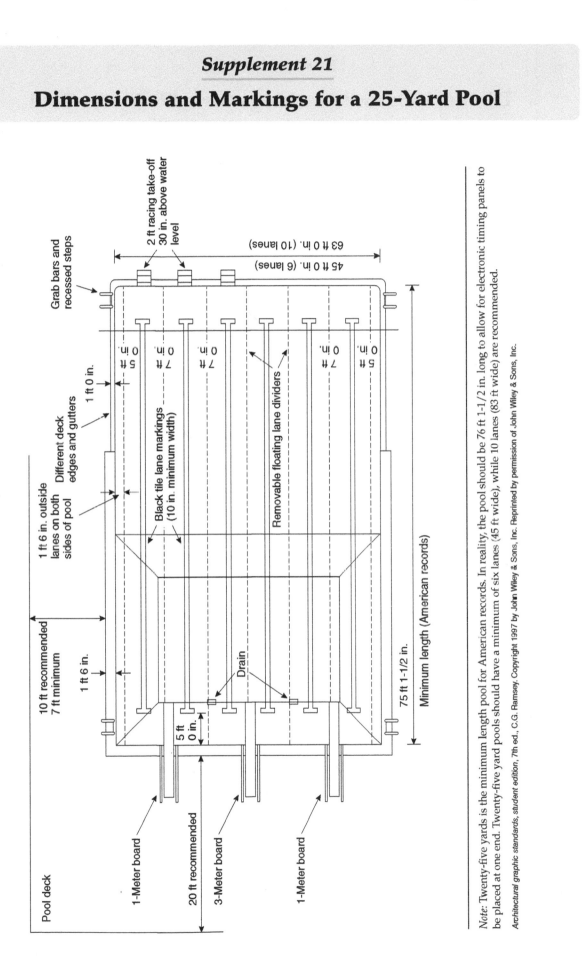

Note: Twenty-five yards is the minimum length pool for American records. In reality, the pool should be 76 ft 1-1/2 in. long to allow for electronic timing panels to be placed at one end. Twenty-five yard pools should have a minimum of six lanes (45 ft wide), while 10 lanes (83 ft wide) are recommended.

Architectural graphic standards, student edition, 7th ed., C.G. Ramsey. Copyright 1997 by John Wiley & Sons, Inc. Reprinted by permission of John Wiley & Sons, Inc.

Supplement 22

Dimensions and Markings for a 50-Meter Pool

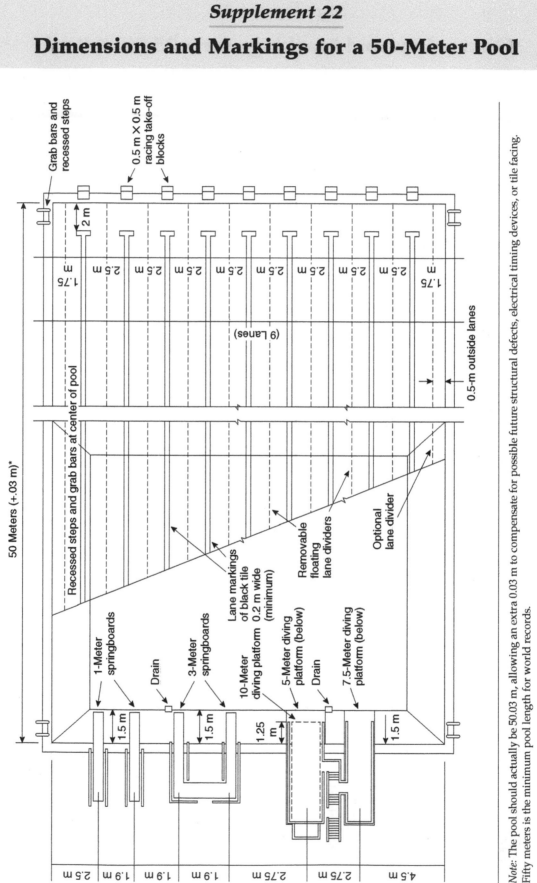

Note: The pool should actually be 50.03 m, allowing an extra 0.03 m to compensate for possible future structural defects, electrical timing devices, or tile facing. Fifty meters is the minimum pool length for world records.

Architectural graphic standards, student edition, 7th ed., C. G. Ramsey, Copyright 1997 by John Wiley & Sons, Inc. Reprinted by permission of John Wiley & Sons, Inc.

Supplement 23

Recommended Diving Pool and Platform Dimensions for Competitive Swimming Programs

Board type	BOARD SIZE			DISTANCES*			
	Length	Width	Height above water level	A From edge of pool to end of board	B From center of board to side of pool	C From center of board to center of board	D From end of board to wall ahead
1-meter springboard	16 ft	20 in.	3 ft 3 in.	A-1 7 ft 5 ft	B-1 10 ft 8 ft	C-1 8 ft 6 ft	D-1 28 ft 25 ft
3-meter springboard	16 ft	20 in.	9 ft 11 in.	A-3 7 ft 5 ft	B-3 15 ft 12 ft	C-3 10 ft 8 ft	D-3 33 ft 30 ft
5-meter platform	18 ft	7 ft	16 ft 5 in.	A-5 7 ft 5 ft	B-5 15 ft 12 ft	C-5 10 ft 8 ft	D-5 43 ft 35 ft
10-meter platform	20 ft 20 ft	8 ft 10 ft	32 ft 10 in.	A-10 8 ft 5 ft	B-10 20 ft 15 ft	C-10 10 ft 8 ft	D-10 52 ft 45 ft

Note: The dimensions in the accompanying table are based upon recommended Olympic requirements. Minimum requirements can be satisfied with a pool 35 ft × 45 ft but a somewhat larger size, for example, 60 ft × 60 ft, is recommended. A water-curling arrangement should be provided so that the diver can see exactly where the surface of the water is. If outdoors, the boards should be oriented so that the sun is not in the diver's eyes. Underwater observation parts are desirable. Diving does not require a very large pool, but it must be deep, with at least a 14-ft depth below a 10-m platform.

*Preferred dimensions appear in the left-hand side of a column, while the minimum safe dimensions are listed in the right-hand side of a column.

Supplement 24

Advantages and Disadvantages
of Selected Types of Pool Overflow Systems

Type	Advantages	Disadvantages
Fully recessed gutter	None	Old-fashioned system Most expensive to build Difficult to clean Contrary to efficient pool operation
Semirecessed gutter	Provides visible pool edge for competition Cuts down surface roughness when gutters are flooded Water surface closer to deck than in fully recessed gutter	Water level 5 or 6 inches below deck; difficult for users to climb out of pool Some cleaning difficulty Requires pipe tunnel for access Narrow edge of gutter lip provides precarious footing for diving off edge
Roll-out gutter	Comfortable pool use and egress Ideal for teaching and recreation Gives beginner swimmers feeling of security by allowing wide visibility Easy cleaning Low construction costs	Decks may flood if adequate number of drains not provided Pool edge not visible for competition; temporary turning boards can be used Requires pipe tunnel for access
Deck-level or rimflow system	Trench serves as integral surge tank Minimum construction costs No pipe tunnel needed Comfortable pool use and egress Ideal for teaching and recreation Gives beginner swimmers feeling of security Easy cleaning	Deck can flood if not properly pitched Pool edge not visible for competition; temporary turning boards can be used Care needed in choosing cleaning materials for deck because some deck water enters pool recirculation system Bottom inlets in rimflow system inaccessible for servicing
Surface skimmers	No surge tank required Suitable for very small pools only	Continuing expense and nuisance of maintaining the moveable weirs Turbulence not eliminated in large pools
Prefabricated stainless steel recessed gutter	Pipe tunnel not required Large diameter return pipe is substituted by the manufacturer for a surge tank	Skimmer weirs need manual adjustments several times a day Waterline inlets disturb swimmers in end lanes Exposed rings for lane and lifelines

Supplement 25

Agencies That Offer Construction Standards for Aquatic Facilities and Associations That Serve the Field of Aquatics

American National Standards Institute
25 W. 43rd Street, 4th floor
New York, NY 10036
212-642-4900
www.ansi.org

American Public Health Association
800 I Street, NW
Washington, DC 20001
202-777-2742
www.apha.org

FINA
Avenue de l'Avante-Poste 4
CH-1005 Lausanne
Switzerland
(+41-21) 310 47 10
www.fina.org

The National Collegiate Athletic Association (NCAA)
700 W. Washington Street
P.O. Box 6222
Indianapolis, IN 46206-6222
317-917-6222
www.ncaa.org

NSF International
789 N. Dixboro Road
P.O. Box 130140
Ann Arbor, MI 48113-0140
800-673-6275
www.nsf.org

National Spas and Pool Institute (NSPI)
2111 Eisenhower Avenue
Alexandria, VA 22314
703-838-0083
www.nspi.org

U.S. Diving
132 E. Washington Street, Suite 850
Indianapolis, IN 46204
317-237-5252
www.usadiving.org

U.S. Swimming
1 Olympic Plaza
Colorado Springs, CO 80909
719-866-4578
www.usaswimming.org

U.S. Synchronized Swimming, Inc.
132 E. Washington Street, Suite 820
Indianapolis, IN 46204
317-237-5700
www.usasynchro.org

Supplement 26

Dimensions and Markings
for a Softball Field for 12-Inch Softball

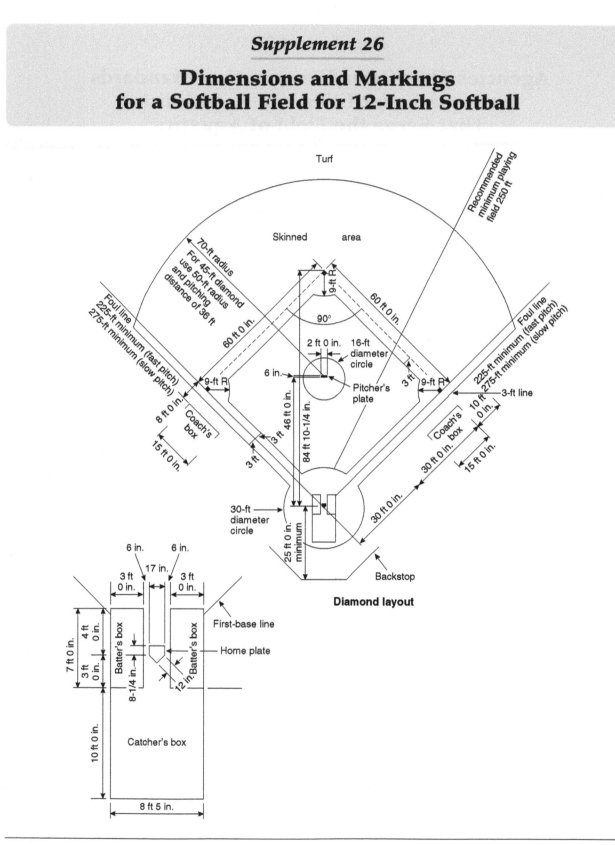

Diamond layout

Note: The recommended baselines are 60 ft for adults and 45 ft for juniors. Distances from home plate to the mound are 46 ft for men, 50 ft for women, and 35 ft for juniors. Juniors should use 45 ft between bases. A field for adult fast-pitch softball should have a 225-ft radius from home plate between the lines. A slow-pitch field has a 275-ft radius and a 250-ft radius for men and women, respectively. The backstop should be located at least 25 ft behind home plate. The foul lines; catcher's, batter's, and coach's boxes; and 3-ft lines should be marked with 2- to 3-in. chalk lines.

Reprinted, by permission, from J. De Chiara and J.H. Callendar, 1990, *Time-saver standards for building types*, 3rd ed. (New York: McGraw-Hill Companies), 1227. © The McGraw-Hill Companies, Inc.

Supplement 27

Dimensions and Markings for a Soccer Field

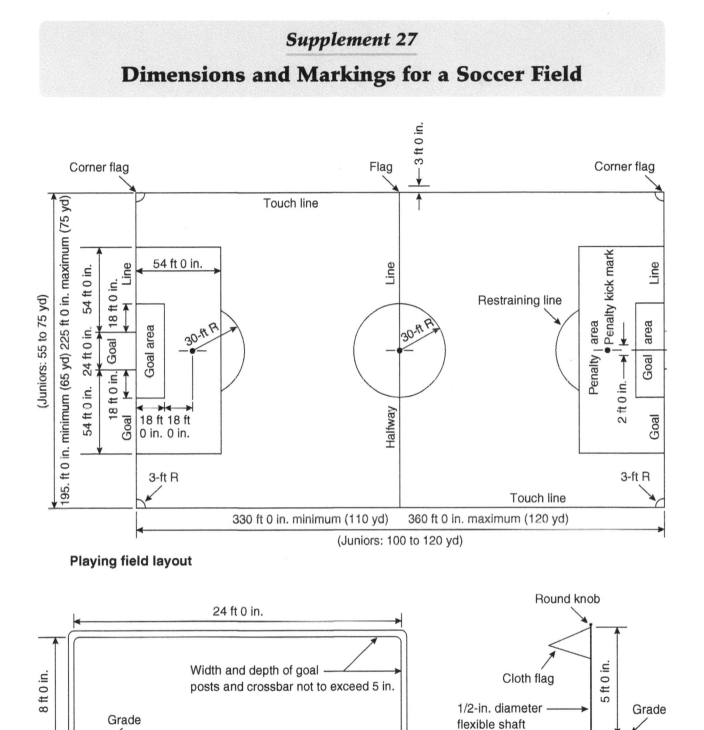

Playing field layout

Goalposts

Flag detail

Note: A full-size soccer field is 195 to 225 ft wide by 330 to 360 ft long, with a minimum unobstructed area of 10 ft on all sides. A soccer field for juniors (and in some instances, women) is usually proportionally smaller. Goalposts should be pressure treated with a paintable, oil-borne preservative and painted above ground with three coats of white lead and oil. The goalposts and crossbar should present a flat surface to the playing field, not less than 4 in. or more than 5 in. in width. Nets should be attached to the posts, crossbar, and ground behind the goal. The top of the net must extend backward 2 ft level with the crossbar. All dimensions are to the inside edge of lines. All lines should be 2 in. wide and marked with a white, nontoxic material that is not injurious to the eyes or skin.

Reprinted, by permission, from J. De Chiara and J.H. Callender, 1990, *Time-saver standards for building types*, 3rd ed. (New York: McGraw-Hill Companies), 1225. © The McGraw-Hill Companies, Inc.

Supplement 28

Playground Equipment Dimensions

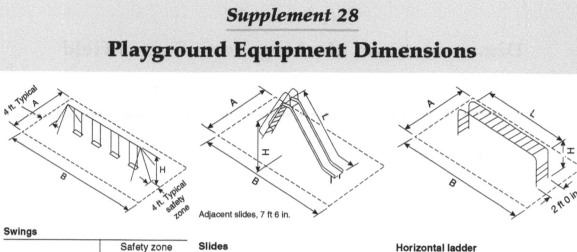

Adjacent slides, 7 ft 6 in.

Swings

Swings	H(ft)	Safety zone A(ft)	Safety zone B(ft)
2	8	24	27
	10	28	27
	12	32	27
3	8	24	30
	10	28	30
	12	32	30
4	8	24	40
	10	28	40
	12	32	40
6	8	24	46
	10	28	46
	12	32	46
8	8	24	57
	10	28	57
	12	32	57
9	8	24	61
	10	28	61
	12	32	61

Slides

H	L	Safety zone A	Safety zone B
4	8	26	24
5	10	26	28
6	12	26	32
8	16	26	36

Horizontal ladder

H (ft, in.)	L (ft, in.)	Safety zone A (ft)	Safety zone B (ft)
6, 6	12, 6	14	25
7, 6	16, 0	14	30

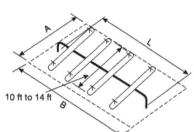

10 ft to 14 ft

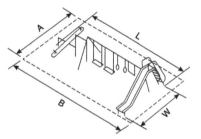

General planning information

Equipment	Area (Sq ft)	Capacity (Number of Children)
Slide	450	4–6
Low swing	150	1
High swing	250	1
Horizontal ladder	375	6–8
Seesaw	100	2
Junior climbing gym	180	8–10
General climbing gym	500	15–20

Seesaws

Boards	1	2	3	4	6
L	3	6	9	12	18
A	20	20	20	20	20
B	5	10	15	20	25

Combination units*

Enclosure limits

A = W + 12 ft 0 in.
B = L + 6 ft 0 in.

*Types and number of units are variable

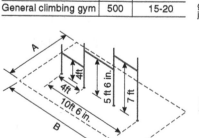

Limits:
A = 8 ft 0 in.
B = L + 6 ft 0 in. heights adjustable

Horizontal bars

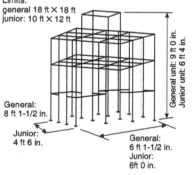

Limits:
general 18 ft × 18 ft
junior: 10 ft × 12 ft

General unit: 9 ft 0 in.
Junior unit: 6 ft 4 in.

General:
8 ft 1-1/2 in.

Junior:
4 ft 6 in.

General:
6 ft 1-1/2 in.
Junior:
6ft 0 in.

N.Y.C. Housing Authority standard climbing gym

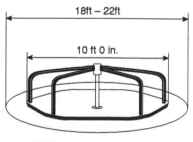

18ft – 22ft

10 ft 0 in.

10 ft diameter is considered standard
Other diameters: 6 ft and 8 ft

Spin around

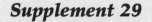

Supplement 29

Outdoor Running Track Lane-Marking Guidelines

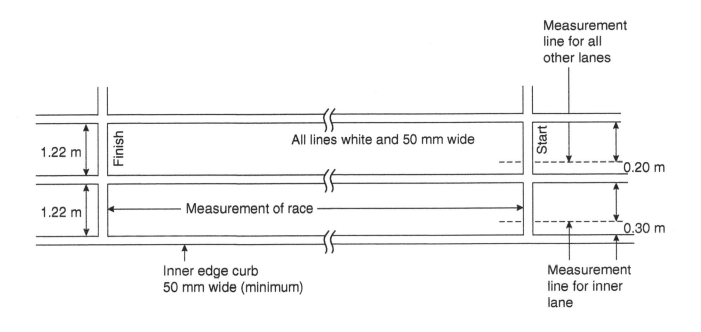

Note: Each lane should be clearly marked and should be a minimum of 1.22 m and a maximum of 1.25 m wide. Each line should be marked by lines 50 mm in width. The inside line of the inside lane should be measured from 0.30 m outward from the inner board of the track. All other lanes should be measured 0.20 m from the outer edge of the preceding line. Tracks used for competition should have a minimum of six lanes; if possible, eight lanes.

Architectural graphic standards, student edition, 7th ed., C.G. Ramsey. Copyright 1997 by John Wiley & Sons, Inc. Reprinted by permission of John Wiley & Sons, Inc.

Supplement 30

Dimensions and Markings for a 440-Yard Running Track

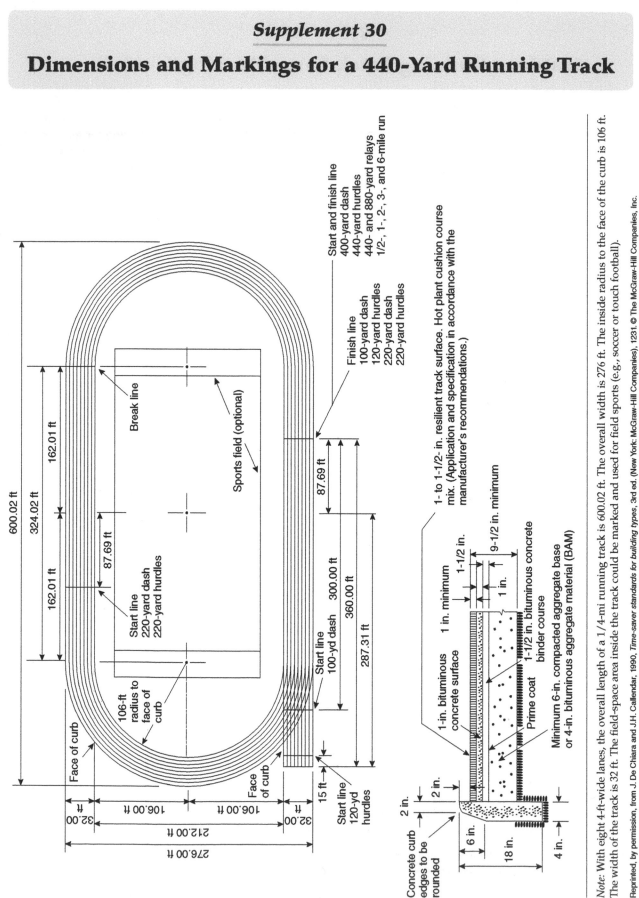

Note: With eight 4-ft-wide lanes, the overall length of a 1/4-mi running track is 600.02 ft. The overall width is 276 ft. The inside radius to the face of the curb is 106 ft. The width of the track is 32 ft. The field-space area inside the track could be marked and used for field sports (e.g., soccer or touch football).

Reprinted, by permission, from J. De Chiara and J.H. Callendar, 1990, *Time-saver standards for building types*, 3rd ed. (New York: McGraw-Hill Companies), 1231. © The McGraw-Hill Companies, Inc.

Supplement 31

Components of a First-Aid Kit

At a minimum, a first-aid kit should contain the following:

- Assorted basic plastic adhesive bandages, various sizes
- 3" × 3" sterile gauze pads (wound dressing)
- 4" × 4" sterile gauze pads (wound dressing)
- 5" × 9" sterile dressing (major wound dressing)
- 3" cohesive bandage (dressing cover)
- Adhesive tape, 2" width (secure dressings, strapping)
- Paper tape, 1" width
- Medical-grade, nonlatex, disposable gloves
- CPR breathing barrier, such as a pocket facemask
- Conforming roller gauze bandage
- Triangular bandages (slings, support, padding)
- Germicidal hand wipes or waterless alcohol-based hand sanitizer
- Antiseptic wipes
- If ice is not immediately available, instant cold packs
- Scissors (first-aid type)
- Tweezers
- Sterile eye pads (emergency eye cover)
- Sterile irrigation solution (wound cleaning, eye wash)
- Emergency blanket
- Current first-aid guide

Supplement 32

AED Prearrival Checklist: Preparing Your Team for AEDs

The following checklist is a quick reference that will help you prepare your employees and members for the arrival of your AED (automated external defibrillator).

____ Review this checklist and the accompanying materials in your AED binder.

____ Pay particular attention to the following sections of this binder, as they will help you the most in preparing for this important program:

- AED policy
- Emergency procedure template
- American Heart Association materials
- AED information
- Support services listing

____ Set up a meeting with your department heads to review the relevant information and discuss your club's strategy (provide handouts of the important information). **During this meeting identify one department head or employee partner to become your AED program coordinator. In addition, discuss how you want to communicate to your members.**

____ Identify the employees who will be part of the initial CPR/AED training. We suggest that these be employees who serve as department heads or employees who cover all of the club's operating hours.

____ Have your AED coordinator set up an AED binder that can be used to store all of the important information, such as the physician's prescription, list of certified employees, weekly operating checklist, AED manual, and club's emergency plan.

____ Have your AED coordinator work with the AED trainer (see the list in your binder) and the AED provider to make sure dates are set up for the training and installation of the program (a calendar of the scheduled training and installation dates will be provided).

____ Establish your club's specific emergency policies so this can be shared with the entire team at a later date.

____ Please note that the AED provider will provide both your physician prescription (standing order) and registration of your AED with the state and local EMS authorities.

____ Arrange a meeting with your entire employee team and share with them the core information about the program and how the club will be implementing the program. Share with them the policies, club emergency plan, proposed member communications, and a list of those who will be receiving training.

____ Arrange to give a presentation to both your board and your committees. Share with them the key information about the program. Discuss with them how to communicate about the AED program to the entire membership.

____ Set up a time line for ongoing training and rehearsal of your program and make it a part of your ongoing operations.

____ Have your AED coordinator make the final arrangements for the training and installation of the club's AED.

Supplement 33

AED Postarrival Checklist:
Creating a Safe Member Environment

This checklist is intended as a quick reference to help you ensure that your team is ready to operate a safe PAD (public access defibrillation) in the club.

____ Make sure that each employee who participates in the AHA Heartsaver AED training receives the proper verification of certification from the AED manager (AHA trainer). Make sure a copy of the certification is placed in the employee's file. You might also consider having a place where you post the names of employees certified in the use and administration of an AED. **Note: You should also place the name of all certified staff in the web-based AED manager program, which will allow you to monitor the club's staff readiness.**

____ Make sure that the AED provider provides your team and your AED coordinator with complete training in the AED functioning before the AED is actually placed in the club. In addition, make sure the AED coordinator has received complete training in the use of the AED manager program. The AED provider will also indicate the best location for your AED.

____ Have your AED coordinator use the AED manager program on a weekly basis. The following are the requirements for use of this program: enter on a weekly or monthly basis the state of readiness of the AED (you will be shown how to do this) and enter the names of all staff who are certified in CPR and AED use and related information that needs to be entered.

____ The AED manager program will e-mail you when it is time for retraining and recertifying staff, when it is time to replace a battery or pad, and when they notice you are not monitoring the equipment as specified. They will also forward automatically at no cost any replacement battery or pads when the system indicates they need to be replaced.

____ Set up an ongoing rehearsal schedule for dealing with emergencies and in particular the administration of the AED. **It is recommended that you hold rehearsals at least once every 6 months. We are providing as part of this program an AED training regimen that allows you to simulate the actual application of the AED. Take advantage of it and rehearse often.**

____ The AED provider is scheduled to make an annual site inspection to test the AED. Make sure that this happens, as it is backup for your weekly and monthly check-ups.

____ If the event you have to use the AED, make sure to follow the guidelines provided in both this binder and in your training as it applies to recording of the event and communicating said event to your designated medical director. You will also need to coordinate the downloading of all event information to the appropriate medical authority. **Please note that the records of any event can be shared only with the medical director overseeing the AED program unless the member or guest indicates in writing otherwise (HIPAA [health insurance portability and accountability act]).**

____ **In the event you have to use the AED, make sure that you immediately complete an incident report and maintain it on file at the club. In addition, complete the event data sheet on the AED manager program, as this will allow immediate communication with AED managers.**

____ Always keep at least two sets of the following on site with your AED: pads, batteries, and rescue kits. When you use one, immediately replace it.

Supplement 34

Public Access Defibrillation Program: Ongoing Readiness Checklist

Monthly Activities the Club Must Perform

- Make sure your club has a designated AED coordinator who is responsible for the program at the club level and is a registered user of the AED manager system.

- The AED coordinator must check the AED readiness status at least once a month by going to the AED and checking the status indicator for a green check. A red X means it is not working.

- The AED coordinator must access the AED manager website for the club at a minimum of once a month. Upon accessing the website, the AED coordinator must do the following:

  ___ Indicate that the AED unit was checked and indicate the status as either working or not (green check indicates it is working, red X means it is not working).

  ___ Update the section for certified AED employees if any certified employee has left the club or if a newly certified employee partner is added.

  ___ Update the AED location section if for some reason the AED has been moved or another AED has been added to the club.

- Review your e-mail for any messages that might be forwarded by the AED manager. The AED manager will e-mail notices when it is time to replace pads or batteries as well as when they notice your AED unit has not been checked.

- When a new employee is hired, make sure that person gets an AED certification within 90 days.

- Have an AED certified employee on duty at the club during all operating hours.

Ongoing Activities (As Needed, Semiannual, and Annual) the Club Must Perform

- Conduct practice AED and emergency drills at least twice a year with your staff.

- Provide refresher AED training at least once a quarter using the practice AED unit and dummy that was provided at the time of your AED installation.

- Maintain the number of AED certified employees on staff at a minimum of 10; when the opportunity arises, make every effort to increase that number.

- Have an annual certification class conducted exclusively by the AED manager. This will ensure that you always have enough certified employees in the club, that a third party has verified the clinical integrity/ readiness of your AED program, and that all on-site information is updated in the AED Manager system.

- In the event your club has an incident that requires the use of the AED, make sure that, after following the proper emergency procedures, you contact the AED manager and complete the incident follow-up procedures within 24 hours.

- Meet with your department heads and other key supervisors at least twice annually to review the various requirements of the program using the AED program information you received at the time of implementation.

- Replace batteries and pads as directed by the AED manager (every two years) or after an incident.

- Maintain an extra battery and set of pads at the club at all times.

Forms

This appendix contains sample forms for use in health and fitness facilities. The law varies from state to state—no form should be adopted or used by any program without individualized legal advice.

1. Physical Activity Readiness Questionnaire (PAR-Q)
2. Health History Questionnaire
3. Guest Health History Questionnaire
4. Physician's Statement and Clearance Form
5. Physician's Approval Form
6. Agreement and Release of Liability Form
7. Informed Consent Agreement
8. Informed Consent for Participation in a Personal Fitness Training Program for Apparently Healthy Adults (Without Known or Suspected Heart Disease)
9. Informed Consent for Exercise Testing of Apparently Healthy Adults (Without Known or Suspected Heart Disease)
10. Informed Consent for Participation in an Exercise Program for Apparently Healthy Adults (Without Known or Suspected Heart Disease)
11. Express Assumption of Risk Form
12. Physician's Release for Activity Form
13. Guest Agreement and Waiver With Brief Medical History
14. Emergency Medical Authorization Form
15. Fitness Evaluation Form
16. Fitness Integration Tracking Form
17. Cardiovascular Assessment Data Sheet
18. Release of Information Form
19. Progress Notes
20. Incident Report Form
21. Theft Report Form
22. Sample Exercise Card
23. Physical Activity Readiness Medical Exam Form (PARmed-X)
24. Emergency Procedures Sheet
25. Health Questionnaire
26. Coronary Risk Factor Identification Form
27. Fitness Testing Form
28. Medical Clearance Form
29. Exercise Contract
30. Health, Fitness, and Racquet Sports Club Incident Report
31. Housekeeping Checklist—Fitness Equipment Room
32. Housekeeping Checklist—Locker Room

Form 1

Physical Activity Readiness Questionnaire
(PAR-Q)

Physical Activity Readiness
Questionnaire - PAR-Q
(revised 2002)

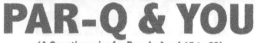

(A Questionnaire for People Aged 15 to 69)

Regular physical activity is fun and healthy, and increasingly more people are starting to become more active every day. Being more active is very safe for most people. However, some people should check with their doctor before they start becoming much more physically active.

If you are planning to become much more physically active than you are now, start by answering the seven questions in the box below. If you are between the ages of 15 and 69, the PAR-Q will tell you if you should check with your doctor before you start. If you are over 69 years of age, and you are not used to being very active, check with your doctor.

Common sense is your best guide when you answer these questions. Please read the questions carefully and answer each one honestly: check YES or NO.

YES	NO		
☐	☐	**1.**	**Has your doctor ever said that you have a heart condition <u>and</u> that you should only do physical activity recommended by a doctor?**
☐	☐	**2.**	**Do you feel pain in your chest when you do physical activity?**
☐	☐	**3.**	**In the past month, have you had chest pain when you were not doing physical activity?**
☐	☐	**4.**	**Do you lose your balance because of dizziness or do you ever lose consciousness?**
☐	☐	**5.**	**Do you have a bone or joint problem (for example, back, knee or hip) that could be made worse by a change in your physical activity?**
☐	☐	**6.**	**Is your doctor currently prescribing drugs (for example, water pills) for your blood pressure or heart condition?**
☐	☐	**7.**	**Do you know of <u>any other reason</u> why you should not do physical activity?**

If

you

answered

YES to one or more questions

Talk with your doctor by phone or in person BEFORE you start becoming much more physically active or BEFORE you have a fitness appraisal. Tell your doctor about the PAR-Q and which questions you answered YES.

- You may be able to do any activity you want — as long as you start slowly and build up gradually. Or, you may need to restrict your activities to those which are safe for you. Talk with your doctor about the kinds of activities you wish to participate in and follow his/her advice.
- Find out which community programs are safe and helpful for you.

NO to all questions

If you answered NO honestly to <u>all</u> PAR-Q questions, you can be reasonably sure that you can:
- start becoming much more physically active — begin slowly and build up gradually. This is the safest and easiest way to go.
- take part in a fitness appraisal — this is an excellent way to determine your basic fitness so that you can plan the best way for you to live actively. It is also highly recommended that you have your blood pressure evaluated. If your reading is over 144/94, talk with your doctor before you start becoming much more physically active.

→

DELAY BECOMING MUCH MORE ACTIVE:
- if you are not feeling well because of a temporary illness such as a cold or a fever — wait until you feel better; or
- if you are or may be pregnant — talk to your doctor before you start becoming more active.

PLEASE NOTE: If your health changes so that you then answer YES to any of the above questions, tell your fitness or health professional. Ask whether you should change your physical activity plan.

<u>Informed Use of the PAR-Q</u>: The Canadian Society for Exercise Physiology, Health Canada, and their agents assume no liability for persons who undertake physical activity, and if in doubt after completing this questionnaire, consult your doctor prior to physical activity.

> **No changes permitted. You are encouraged to photocopy the PAR-Q but only if you use the entire form.**

NOTE: If the PAR-Q is being given to a person before he or she participates in a physical activity program or a fitness appraisal, this section may be used for legal or administrative purposes.

"I have read, understood and completed this questionnaire. Any questions I had were answered to my full satisfaction."

NAME _____

SIGNATURE _____ DATE _____

SIGNATURE OF PARENT _____ WITNESS _____
or GUARDIAN (for participants under the age of majority)

> **Note: This physical activity clearance is valid for a maximum of 12 months from the date it is completed and becomes invalid if your condition changes so that you would answer YES to any of the seven questions.**

CSEP
SCPE © Canadian Society for Exercise Physiology   Supported by: ✚ Health   Santé
                                                          Canada Canada   continued on other side...

Form 2

Health History Questionnaire

Name _____ Company _____

Home address _____

Position _____

Telephone (home) _____ (work) _____

Height _____ Weight _____

Gender _____ Birth date _____ Age _____

Regular physical activity is safe for most people. However, some individuals should check with their doctor before they start an exercise program. To help us determine if you should consult with your doctor before starting to exercise with (your organization), please read the following questions carefully and answer each one honestly. All information will be kept confidential. Please check YES or NO:

YES NO

☐ ☐   1. Do you have a heart condition?

☐ ☐   2. Have you ever experienced a stroke?

☐ ☐   3. Do you have epilepsy?

☐ ☐   4. Are you pregnant?

☐ ☐   5. Do you have diabetes?

☐ ☐   6. Do you have emphysema?

☐ ☐   7. Do you feel pain in your chest when you engage in physical activity?

☐ ☐   8. Do you have chronic bronchitis?

☐ ☐   9. In the past month, have you had chest pain when you were not doing physical activity?

☐ ☐ 10. Do you ever lose consciousness or do you ever lose control of your balance due to chronic dizziness?

☐ ☐ 11. Are you currently being treated for a bone or joint problem that restricts you from engaging in physical activity?

☐ ☐ 12. Has a physician ever told you or are you aware that you have high blood pressure?

☐ ☐ 13. Has anyone in your immediate family (parents/brothers/sisters) had a heart attack, stroke, or cardiovascular disease before age 55?

☐ ☐ 14. Has a physician ever told you or are you aware that you have a high cholesterol level?

☐ ☐ 15. Do you currently smoke?

☐ ☐ 16. Are you a male over 44 years of age?

☐ ☐ 17. Are you a female over 54 years of age?

☐ ☐ 18. Are you currently exercising *LESS* than 1 hour per week? If you answered no, please list your activities.

_____

☐ ☐ 19. Are you currently taking any medication?

Please list the medication and its purpose _____

(continued)

(continued)

What are your specific fitness goals at (your organization)? (Indicate all that apply)

☐ Increase strength and endurance	☐ Improve flexibility
☐ Improve cardiovascular fitness	☐ Improve muscle tone
☐ Reduce body fat	☐ Increase muscle mass
☐ Exercise regularly	☐ Injury rehabilitation
☐ Sports conditioning	☐ Other _____

What are your specific health goals at (your organization)? (Indicate all that apply)

☐ Reduce stress	☐ Improve nutritional habits
☐ Control blood pressure	☐ Control cholesterol
☐ Stop smoking	☐ Achieve balance in life
☐ Improve productivity	☐ Reduce back pain
☐ Feel better overall	☐ Increase my health awareness

☐ Other (please be specific) _____

What motivated you to join (your organization)? (Indicate all that apply)

☐ Convenience/location

☐ Membership promotion

☐ Attended a (your organization) health promotion event at work

☐ Peer support

☐ Medical reasons

☐ Tried (your organization) as a guest

☐ Corporate membership

☐ Other _____

I have read, understood, and completed this questionnaire. Any questions that I had were answered to my full satisfaction.

Name _____ Date _____

Signature _____

STAFF USE ONLY

Cleared to exercise _____ **Not cleared to exercise** _____

Reason _____

Staff Signature _____ **Date** _____

Resting Heart Rate _____

Resting Blood Pressure _____

EP _____

Form 3

Guest Health History Questionnaire

Name _____ Date _____

Date of birth _____

Employer _____

Title _____

Home address _____ City _____ Zip _____

Phone (home) _____ (work) _____

Gender (Please circle)   M   F

Guest of _____

Health insurance provider _____

In case of emergency contact _____

Regular physical activity is safe for most people. However, some individuals should check with their doctor before they start an exercise program. To help us determine if you should consult with your doctor before starting to exercise with (your organization), please read the following questions carefully and answer each one honestly. All information will be kept confidential. Please check YES or NO:

YES NO

☐ ☐   1. Do you have a heart condition?

☐ ☐   2. Have you ever experienced a stroke?

☐ ☐   3. Do you have epilepsy?

☐ ☐   4. Are you pregnant?

☐ ☐   5. Do you have diabetes?

☐ ☐   6. Do you have emphysema?

☐ ☐   7. Do you feel pain in your chest when you engage in physical activity?

☐ ☐   8. Do you have chronic bronchitis?

☐ ☐   9. In the past month, have you had chest pain when you were not doing physical activity?

☐ ☐ 10. Do you ever lose consciousness or do you ever lose control of your balance due to chronic dizziness?

☐ ☐ 11. Are you currently being treated for a bone or joint problem that restricts you from engaging in physical activity?

☐ ☐ 12. Has a physician ever told you or are you aware that you have high blood pressure?

☐ ☐ 13. Has anyone in your immediate family (parents/brothers/sisters) had a heart attack, stroke, or cardiovascular disease before age 55?

☐ ☐ 14. Has a physician ever told you or are you aware that you have a high cholesterol level?

☐ ☐ 15. Do you currently smoke?

(continued)

(continued)

YES NO

☐ ☐ 16. Are you a male over 44 years of age?

☐ ☐ 17. Are you a female over 54 years of age?

☐ ☐ 18. Are you currently exercising *LESS* than 1 hour per week? If you answered no, please list your activities.

_____

☐ ☐ 19. Are you currently taking any medication? Please list the medication and its purpose.

_____

How did you hear about (your organization)?

_____ Employer   _____ Yellow Pages   _____ Friend

_____ Television   _____ Newspaper   _____ Radio

_____ Co-worker   _____ Health ins. plan   _____ Worksite event

Are you interested in joining (your organization)?   Y or N

Are you interested in learning how (your organization) can develop a corporate fitness and wellness benefit for your organization?   Y or N

I understand that any exercise program I undertake may create physical stress and subsequent harmful effects. I agree that it is solely my responsibility and not the responsibility of (your organization) to require me to consult with a physician prior to commencing any exercise program, to remain under medical supervision if that is indicated, and to seek medical assistance in the event of an injury. I recognize that the use of the equipment entails some risk of accidental injury to myself and to others and I agree that I will use such equipment and facilities with due care.

Signature _____   Date _____

STAFF USE ONLY

☐ Cleared to exercise   ☐ Not cleared to exercise   ☐ Guest # _____

Reason _____

Staff Signature _____   Date _____

Visit Date/Time _____   Visit Date/Time _____

Visit Date/Time _____   Visit Date/Time _____

Visit Date/Time _____   Visit Date/Time _____

Form 4

Physician's Statement and Clearance Form

At (your organization), your safety is our primary concern. For that reason, we comply with the health and fitness standards of the American College of Sports Medicine and the International Health, Racquet and Sportsclub Association.

On the Health History Questionnaire you just completed, you identified that you have one or more coronary and/or other medical risk factors that may impair your ability to exercise safely. For this reason, you need to have a physician complete and return this medical clearance form before you can begin exercising at (your organization).

We recognize that you are eager to start your fitness program, and we sincerely regret any inconvenience that this may cause you. However, please keep in mind that we want your exercise experience at (your organization) to be as safe as possible.

In order to expedite this process, we will gladly fax this form directly to the physician of your choice. If the doctor is aware of your medical history, he/she may be able to complete this form and fax it right back to us. In many cases the delay is only one day.

I hereby give my physician permission to release any pertinent medical information from any medical records to the staff at (your organization). All information will be kept confidential.

Patient's signature _____ Date _____

Information requested for _____

Reason for medical clearance _____

Physician's name _____

Phone _____ Fax _____

Address _____

For Physician Use Only

Please check one of the following statements:

_____ I concur with my patient's participation with no restrictions.

_____ I concur with my patient's participation in an exercise program if he/she restricts activities to:

_____

_____ I do not concur with my patient's participation in an exercise program
(if checked, the individual will not be allowed to join [your organization]).

Reason _____

Physician's name (type or print) _____

Physician's signature _____ Date _____

Please return fax to: General Manager _____

Phone _____ **Fax** _____

Form 5

Physician's Approval Form

_____ has medical approval to participate in fitness programs and in the use of exercise equipment at various sites, including home or office, that may be provided by and/or recommended by _____ .

The following restrictions apply (if none, so state): _____

_____

_____

_____

_____

_____
Physician's signature

_____
Physician's name

_____
Street address

_____ _____ _____
City   State   Zip

_____
Phone

_____
Date

*** Please attach a copy of the results of the latest physical examination.

Form 6

Agreement and Release of Liability Form

1. In consideration of gaining membership or being allowed to participate in the activities and programs of _____ and to use its facilities, equipment, and machinery in addition to the payment of any fee or charge, I do hereby waive, release and forever discharge _____ and its officers, agents, employees, representatives, executors, and all others from any and all responsibilities or liability for injuries or damages resulting from my participation in any activities or my use of equipment or machinery in the above-mentioned facilities or arising out of my participation in any activities at said facility. I do also hereby release all of those mentioned and any others acting upon their behalf from any responsibility or liability for any injury or damage to myself, including those caused by the negligent act or omission of any of those mentioned or others acting on their behalf or in any way arising out of or connected with my participation in any activities of _____ or the use of any equipment at _____ . (**Please initial** _____)

2. I understand and am aware that strength, feasibility, and aerobic exercise, including the use of equipment, is a potentially hazardous activity. I also understand that fitness activities involve a risk of injury and even death and that I am voluntarily participating in these activities and using equipment and machinery with knowledge of the dangers involved. I hereby agree to expressly assume and accept any and all risks of injury or death. (**Please initial** _____)

3. I do hereby further declare myself to be physically sound and suffering from no condition, impairment, disease, infirmity, or other illness that would prevent my participation in any of the activities and programs of _____ or use of equipment or machinery except as hereinafter stated. I do hereby acknowledge that I have been informed of the need for a physician's approval for my participation in an exercise/fitness activity or in the use of exercise equipment and machinery. I also acknowledge that it has been recommended that I have a yearly or more frequent physical examination and consultation with my physician as to physical activity, exercise, and use of exercise and training equipment so that I might have recommendations concerning these fitness activities and equipment use. I acknowledge that I have either had a physical examination and have been given a physician's permission to participate, or that I have decided to participate in activity and/or use of equipment and machinery without the approval of my physician and do hereby assume all responsibility for my participation and activities, and utilization of equipment and machinery in my activities. (**Please initial** _____)

Date _____ Signature _____

Note: The law varies from state to state. No form should be adopted or used by any program without individualized legal advice.

Reprinted, by permission, from D. Herbert, 1989, "Avoiding allegations of misrepresentation/fraud in program documents," *The Exercise Standards and Malpractice Reporter* 3(2): 30-31.

Form 7

Informed Consent Agreement

Thank you for choosing to use the facilities, services, or programs of _____. We request your understanding and cooperation in maintaining both your and our safety and health by reading and signing the following informed consent agreement.

I, _____, declare that I intend to use some or all of the activities, facilities, programs, and services offered by _____ and I understand that each person, myself included, has a different capacity for participating in such activities, facilities, programs, and services. I am aware that all activities, services, and programs offered are either educational, recreational, or self-directed in nature. I assume full responsibility, during and after my participation, for my choices to use or apply, at my own risk, any portion of the information or instruction I receive.

I understand that part of the risk involved in undertaking any activity or program is relative to my own state of fitness or health (physical, mental, or emotional) and to the awareness, care, and skill with which I conduct myself in that activity or program. I acknowledge that my choice to participate in any activity, service, and program of _____ brings with it my assumption of those risks or results stemming from this choice and the fitness, health, awareness, care, and skill that I possess and use.

I further understand that the activities, programs, and services offered by _____ are sometimes conducted by personnel who may not be licensed, certified, or registered instructors or professionals. I accept the fact that the skills and competencies of some employees and/or volunteers will vary according to their training and experience and that no claim is made to offer assessment or treatment of any mental or physical disease or condition by those who are not duly licensed, certified, or registered and herein employed to provide such professional services.

I recognize that by participating in the activities, facilities, programs, and services offered by _____, I may experience potential health risks such as transient light-headedness, fainting, abnormal blood pressure, chest discomfort, leg cramps, and nausea and that I assume willfully those risks. I acknowledge my obligation to immediately inform the nearest supervising employee of any pain, discomfort, fatigue, or any other symptoms that I may suffer during and immediately after my participation. I understand that I may stop or delay my participation in any activity or procedure if I so desire and that I may also be requested to stop and rest by a supervising employee who observes any symptoms of distress or abnormal response.

I understand that I may ask any questions or request further explanation or information about the activities, facilities, programs, and services offered by _____ at any time before, during, or after my participation.

I declare that I have read, understood, and agree to the contents of this informed consent agreement in its entirety.

Signature _____

Date of signing _____

Witness _____

Note: The law varies from state to state. No form should be adopted or used by any program without individualized legal advice.

Adapted, by permission, from D. Herbert, 1994, *Legal aspects of sports medicine,* 2nd ed. (Canton, OH: Professional Reports Corporation).

Informed Consent for Participation in a Personal Fitness Training Program for Apparently Healthy Adults

(Without Known or Suspected Heart Disease)

Name _____

1. PURPOSE AND EXPLANATION OF PROCEDURE

I hereby consent to voluntarily engage in an acceptable plan of personal fitness training. I also give consent to be placed in personal fitness training program activities that are recommended to me for improvement of my general health and well-being. These may include dietary counseling, stress management, and health/fitness education activities. The levels of exercise I perform will be based on my cardiorespiratory (heart and lungs) and muscular fitness. I understand that I may be required to undergo a graded exercise test as well as other fitness tests prior to the start of my personal fitness training program in order to evaluate and assess my present level of fitness. I will be given exact personal instructions regarding the amount and kind of exercise I should do. I agree to participate 3 times per week in the formal program sessions. Professionally trained personal fitness trainers will provide leadership to direct my activities, monitor my performance, and otherwise evaluate my effort. Depending on my health status, I may or may not be required to have my blood pressure and heart rate evaluated during these sessions to regulate my exercise within desired limits. I understand that I am expected to attend every session and to follow staff instructions with regard to exercise, diet, stress management, and other health/fitness-related programs. If I am taking prescribed medications, I have already so informed the program staff and further agree to so inform them promptly of any changes my doctor or I make with regard to use of these. I will be given the opportunity for periodic assessment and evaluation at regular intervals after the start of my program.

I have been informed that during my participation in this personal fitness training program, I will be asked to complete the physical activities unless symptoms such as fatigue, shortness of breath, chest discomfort, or similar occurrences appear. At that point, I have been advised that it is my complete right to decrease or stop exercise and that it is my obligation to inform the personal fitness training program personnel of my symptoms. I hereby state that I have been so advised and agree to inform the personal fitness training program personnel of my symptoms, should any develop.

I understand that while I exercise, a personal fitness trainer will periodically monitor my performance and perhaps measure my pulse and blood pressure or assess my feelings of effort for the purposes of monitoring my progress. I also understand that the personal fitness trainer may reduce or stop my exercise program when any of these findings so indicate that this should be done for my safety and benefit.

I also understand that during the performance of my personal fitness training program, physical touching and positioning of my body may be necessary to assess my muscular and bodily reactions to specific exercises, as well as ensure that I am using proper technique and body alignment. I expressly consent to the physical contact for these reasons.

2. RISKS

I understand and have been informed that there exists the remote possibility of adverse changes occurring during exercise including, but not limited to, abnormal blood pressure, fainting, dizziness, disorders of heart rhythm, and very rare instances of heart attack, stroke, or even death. I further understand and I have been informed that there exists the risk of bodily injury including, but not limited to, injuries to the muscles, ligaments, tendons, and joints of the body. I have been told that every effort will be made to minimize these occurrences by proper staff assessments of my condition before each exercise session, by staff supervision

(continued)

(continued)

during exercise, and by my own careful control of exercise efforts. I fully understand the risks associated with exercise, including the risk of bodily injury, heart attack, stroke, or even death, but knowing these risks, it is my desire to participate as herein indicated.

3. BENEFITS TO BE EXPECTED AND AVAILABLE ALTERNATIVES TO EXERCISE

I understand that this program may or may not benefit my physical fitness or general health. I recognize that involvement in the exercise sessions and personal fitness training sessions will allow me to learn proper ways to perform conditioning exercises, use fitness equipment, and regulate physical effort. These experiences should benefit me by indicating how my physical limitations may affect my ability to perform various physical activities. I further understand that if I closely follow the program's instructions, I will likely improve my exercise capacity and fitness level after a period of 3 to 6 months.

4. CONFIDENTIALITY AND USE OF INFORMATION

I have been informed that the information obtained in this personal fitness training program will be treated as privileged and confidential and will consequently not be released or revealed to any person without my express written consent. I do, however, agree to the use of any information that is not personally identifiable with me for research and statistical purposes so long as same does not identify me or provide facts that could lead to my identification. I also agree to the use of any information for the purpose of consultation with other health/fitness professionals, including my doctor. Any other information obtained, however, will be used by the program staff in the course of prescribing exercise for me and evaluating my progress in the program.

5. INQUIRIES AND FREEDOM OF CONSENT

I have been given an opportunity to ask certain questions as to the procedures of this program. Generally, these requests have been noted by the interviewing staff with his/her responses as follows:

_____

_____

_____

I further understand that there are also other remote risks that may be associated with this personal fitness training program. Despite the fact that a complete accounting of all these remote risks has not been provided to me, it is still my desire to participate.

I acknowledge that I have read this document in its entirety or that it has been read to me if I have been unable to read same.

I expressly consent to the rendition of all services and procedures as explained herein by all program personnel.

Date _____

_____
Client's signature

By _____
Authorized representative

Note: The law varies from state to state. No form should be adopted or used by any program without individualized legal advice.

Reprinted, by permission, from B.E. Koeberle, 1990, *Legal aspects of personal fitness training* (Canton, OH: Professional Reports Corporation), 149-151.

Form 9

Informed Consent for Exercise Testing of Apparently Healthy Adults

(Without Known or Suspected Heart Disease)

Name _____

1. PURPOSE AND EXPLANATION OF TEST

I hereby consent to voluntarily engage in an exercise test to determine my circulatory and respiratory fitness. I also consent to the taking of samples of my exhaled air during exercise to properly measure my oxygen consumption. I also consent, if necessary, to have a small blood sample drawn by needle from my arm for blood chemistry analysis and to the performance of lung function and body fat (skinfold pinch) tests. It is my understanding that the information obtained will help me evaluate future physical activities and sports activities in which I may engage.

Before I undergo the test, I certify to the program that I am in good health and have had a physical examination conducted by a licensed medical physician within the last _____ months. Further, I hereby represent and inform the program that I have completed the pretest history interview presented to me by the program staff and have provided correct responses to the questions as indicated on the history form or as supplied to the interviewer. It is my understanding that I will be interviewed by a physician or other person prior to my undergoing the test who will in the course of interviewing me determine if there are any reasons which would make it undesirable or unsafe for me to take the test. Consequently, I understand that it is important that I provide complete and accurate responses to the interviewer and recognize that my failure to do so could lead to possible unnecessary injury to myself during the test.

The test I will undergo will be performed on a motor-driven treadmill or bicycle ergometer with the amount of effort gradually increasing. As I understand it, this increase in effort will continue until I feel and verbally report to the operator any symptoms such as fatigue, shortness of breath, or chest discomfort which may appear. It is my understanding and I have been clearly advised that it is my right to request that a test be stopped at any point if I feel unusual discomfort or fatigue. I have been advised that I should immediately upon experiencing any such symptoms, or if I so choose, inform the operator that I wish to stop the test at that or any other point. My wishes in this regard shall be absolutely carried out.

It is further my understanding that prior to beginning the test, I will be connected by electrodes and cables to an electrocardiographic recorder, which will enable the program personnel to monitor my cardiac (heart) activity. It is my understanding that during the test itself, a trained observer will monitor my responses continuously and take frequent readings of blood pressure, the electrocardiogram, and my expressed feelings of effort. I realize that a true determination of my exercise capacity depends on progressing the test to the point of my fatigue.

Once the test has been completed, but before I am released from the test area, I will be given special instructions about showering and recognition of certain symptoms that may appear within the first 24 hours after the test. I agree to follow these instructions and promptly contact the program personnel or medical providers if such symptoms develop.

2. RISKS

I understand and have been informed that there exists the possibility of adverse changes during the actual test. I have been informed that these changes could include abnormal blood pressure, fainting, disorders of heart rhythm, stroke, and very rare instances of heart attack or even death. I have been told that every effort

(continued)

(continued)

will be made to minimize these occurrences by preliminary examination and by precautions and observations taken during the test. I have also been informed that emergency equipment and personnel are readily available to deal with these unusual situations should they occur. I understand that there is a risk of injury, heart attack, or even death as a result of my performance of this test, but knowing those risks, it is my desire to proceed to take the test as herein indicated.

3. BENEFITS TO BE EXPECTED AND AVAILABLE ALTERNATIVES TO THE EXERCISE TESTING PROCEDURE

The results of this test may or may not benefit me. Potential benefits relate mainly to my personal motives for taking the test, that is, knowing my exercise capacity in relation to the general population, understanding my fitness for certain sports and recreational activities, planning my physical conditioning program, or evaluating the effects of my recent physical activity habits. Although my fitness might also be evaluated by alternative means, for example, a bench step test or an outdoor running test, such tests do not provide as accurate a fitness assessment as the treadmill or bike test nor do those options allow equally effective monitoring of my responses.

4. CONFIDENTIALITY AND USE OF INFORMATION

I have been informed that the information obtained in this exercise test will be treated as privileged and confidential and will consequently not be released or revealed to any person without my express written consent. I do, however, agree to the use of any information for research or statistical purposes so long as same does not provide facts that could lead to my identification. Any other information obtained, however, will be used only by the program staff to evaluate my exercise status or needs.

5. INQUIRIES AND FREEDOM OF CONSENT

I have been given an opportunity to ask certain questions as to the procedures. Generally these requests, which have been noted by the testing staff, and their responses are as follows:

_____

_____

_____

I further understand that there are also other remote risks that may be associated with this procedure. Despite the fact that a complete accounting of all these remote risks has not been provided to me, I still desire to proceed with the test.

I acknowledge that I have read this document in its entirety or that it has been read to me if I have been unable to read same.

I consent to the rendition of all services and procedures as explained herein by all program personnel.

Date _____

_____

Participant's signature

_____

Witness' signature

_____

Test supervisor's signature

_____

Note: The law varies from state to state. No form should be adopted or used by any program without individualized legal advice.

Reprinted, by permission, from D. Herbert, 1994, *Legal aspects of sports medicine*, 2nd ed. (Canton, OH: Professional Reports Corporation).

Form 10

Informed Consent for Participation in an Exercise Program for Apparently Healthy Adults

(Without Known or Suspected Heart Disease)

Name _____

1. PURPOSE AND EXPLANATION OF PROCEDURE

I hereby consent to voluntarily engage in an acceptable plan of exercise conditioning. I also give consent to be placed in program activities that are recommended to me for improvement of my general health and well-being. These may include dietary counseling, stress reduction, and health education activities. The levels of exercise I will perform will be based upon my cardiorespiratory (heart and lungs) fitness as determined through my recent laboratory graded exercise evaluation. I will be given exact instructions regarding the amount and kind of exercise I should do. I agree to participate 3 times per week in the formal program sessions. Professionally trained personnel will provide leadership to direct my activities, monitor my performance, and otherwise evaluate my effort. Depending upon my health status, I may or may not be required to have my blood pressure and heart rate evaluated during these sessions to regulate my exercise within desired limits. I understand that I am expected to attend every session and to follow staff instructions with regard to exercise, diet, stress management, and smoking cessation. If I am taking prescribed medications, I have already so informed the program staff and further agree to so inform them promptly of any changes my doctor or I make with regard to use of these. I will be given the opportunity for periodic assessment with laboratory evaluations at 6 months after the start of my program. Should I remain in the program thereafter, additional evaluations will generally be given at 12 month intervals. The program may change the foregoing schedule of evaluations, if this is considered desirable for health reasons.

I have been informed that during my participation in exercise, I will be asked to complete the physical activities unless symptoms such as fatigue, shortness of breath, chest discomfort, or similar occurrences appear. At that point, I have been advised it is my complete right to decrease or stop exercise and that it is my obligation to inform the program personnel of my symptoms. I hereby state that I have been so advised and agree to inform the program personnel of my symptoms, should any develop.

I understand that, while I exercise, a trained observer will periodically monitor my performance and perhaps measure my pulse and blood pressure or assess my feelings of effort for the purposes of monitoring my progress. I also understand that the observer may reduce or stop my exercise program when any of these findings so indicate that this should be done for my safety and benefit.

2. RISKS

I understand and have been informed that there exists the remote possibility during exercise of adverse changes including abnormal blood pressure, fainting, disorders of heart rhythm, and very rare instances of heart attack or even death. I have been told that every effort will be made to minimize these occurrences by proper staff assessment of my condition before each exercise session, by staff supervision during exercise, and by my own careful control of exercise efforts. I have also been informed that emergency equipment and personnel are readily available to deal with unusual situations should these occur. I understand that there is a risk of injury, heart attack, or even death as a result of my exercise, but knowing those risks, I desire to participate as herein indicated.

(continued)

(continued)

3. BENEFITS TO BE EXPECTED AND ALTERNATIVES AVAILABLE TO EXERCISE

I understand that this program may or may not benefit my physical fitness or general health. I recognize that involvement in the exercise sessions will allow me to learn proper ways to perform conditioning exercises, use fitness equipment, and regulate physical effort. These experiences should benefit me by indicating how my physical limitations may affect my ability to perform various physical activities. I further understand that if I closely follow the program instructions, I will likely improve my exercise capacity after a period of 3 to 6 months.

4. CONFIDENTIALITY AND USE OF INFORMATION

I have been informed that the information obtained in this exercise program will be treated as privileged and confidential and will consequently not be released or revealed to any person without my express written consent. I do, however, agree to the use of any information that is not personally identifiable with me for research and statistical purposes so long as same does not identify me or provide facts that could lead to my identification. Any other information obtained, however, will be used only by the program staff in the course of prescribing exercise for me and evaluating my progress in the program.

5. INQUIRIES AND FREEDOM OF CONSENT

I have been given an opportunity to ask certain questions as to the procedures of this program. Generally these requests have been noted by the interviewing staff member, and his/her responses are as follows.

_____

_____

_____

I further understand that there are also other remote risks that may be associated with this program. Despite the fact that a complete accounting of all these remote risks has not been provided to me, I still desire to participate.

I acknowledge that I have read this document in its entirety or that it has been read to me if I have been unable to read same.

I consent to the rendition of all services and procedures as explained herein by all program personnel.

Date _____

_____
Participant's signature

_____
Witness' signature

_____
Test supervisor's signature

Note: The law varies from state to state. No form should be adopted or used by any program without individualized legal advice.

Reprinted, by permission, from D. Herbert, 1994, *Legal aspects of sports medicine*, 2nd ed. (Canton, OH: Professional Reports Corporation).

Form 11

Express Assumption of Risk Form

I, the undersigned, hereby expressly and affirmatively state that I wish to participate in _____.
I realize that my participation in this activity involves risks of injury, including but not limited to _____
(list) _____ and even the possibility of death. I also recognize that there are many other risks of injury,
including serious disabling injuries, that may arise due to my participation in this activity and that it is not
possible to specifically list each and every individual injury risk. However, knowing the material risks and
appreciating, knowing, and reasonably anticipating that other injuries and even death are a possibility, I
hereby expressly assume all of the delineated risks of injury, all other possible risk of injury, and even risk
of death, which could occur by reason of my participation.

I have had an opportunity to ask questions. Any questions I have asked have been answered to my
complete satisfaction. I subjectively understand the risks of my participation in this activity, and knowing
and appreciating these risks, I voluntarily choose to participate, assuming all risks of injury or even death
due to my participation.

_____   _____
Witness   Participant

_____
Dated

Notes of questions and answers

_____

_____

_____

This is, as stated, a true and accurate record of what was asked and answered.

_____
Participant

To be checked by program staff	*Checked*	*Initials*
I. Risks were orally discussed.	_____	_____
II. Questions were asked, and the participant indicated complete understanding of the risks.	_____	_____
III. Questions were not asked, but an opportunity to ask questions was provided and the participant indicated complete understanding of the risks.	_____	_____

_____   _____
Staff member   Dated

Note: The law varies from state to state. No form should be adopted or used by any program without individualized legal advice.

Form 12

Physician's Release for Activity Form

_____ has recently enrolled for membership at East Side/West Side Athletic Clubs. The club membership includes two complimentary orientation sessions with our qualified fitness professionals (degreed and/or certified in the field), as well as the opportunity to participate in numerous group fitness classes and individual programs.

On completion of the PAR-Q (Physical Activity Readiness Questionnaire), it has been determined that this new member is best served by additional or supplemental recommendations by his/her care provider.

Please take the time to review your client's medical history and the PAR-Q accompanied with this request. If he/she can be released for physical activity, please complete the information below and let us know if there are any modifications or special needs.

Member's signature for release of information _____

Date _____

Club staff faxing this information (print name) _____

As a physician, it is my understanding that the person listed above wishes to participate in physical activity at the Club and has been referred to myself (his/her physician) before beginning a regular program. **Here are my specific recommendations and/or comments regarding this new member and his/her involvement in an exercise program:**

Physician's printed name _____

Date _____

Physician's signature _____

Form 13

Guest Agreement and Waiver With Brief Medical History

Date _____

Name _____

Company name _____

Mailing address _____

City _____ State _____ Zip _____

Phone: (W) _____ (H) _____

Guest of: _____

Please answer the following seven questions

YES NO

☐ ☐ 1. Has your doctor ever said you have heart trouble?

☐ ☐ 2. Do you frequently have pains in your heart and chest?

☐ ☐ 3. Do you often feel faint or have spells of severe dizziness?

☐ ☐ 4. Has a doctor ever said your blood pressure was too high?

☐ ☐ 5. Has your doctor ever told you that you have a bone or joint problem such as arthritis that has been aggravated by exercise or might be made worse by exercise?

☐ ☐ 6. Is there any good physical reason not mentioned here why you should not follow an activity program even if you wanted to?

☐ ☐ 7. Are you over age 65 and not accustomed to vigorous exercise?

Guest Agreement/Waiver

The undersigned guest agrees to abide by the rules of the Club, including the completion of the above medical questionnaire.

The undersigned guest agrees that all use of the Club's facilities, services and programs shall be undertaken at his/her sole risk and the Club shall not be liable for any injuries, accidents or deaths occurring to guest, arising either directly or indirectly out of utilizing the Club's facilities, services and programs. The guest, for him/herself and on behalf of his/her executors, administrators, heirs, and assigns, does hereby expressly release, discharge, waive, relinquish, and covenant not to sue the Club, its officers, and agents for all such claims, demands, injuries, damages, or causes of action, with respect to use of the Club's facilities, programs, and services.

The undersigned guest declares that he/she has completed the enclosed medical questionnaire as required by the Club and that he/she declares he/she is physically able to participate in physical activity. Furthermore, guest declares that the Club has advised guest to obtain a medical clearance in the event he/she answer yes to any of the medical history questions, or if he/she is unsure of his/her physical health and that guest maintains that he/she is physically capable of pursuing physical activity in the Club without such steps being taken or has done so.

Guest signature _____

Date _____

Form 14

Emergency Medical Authorization Form

I/we, the undersigned, am/are the father and mother of _____ minor(s).

CONSENT

I/we hereby give consent, in the event I/we cannot be contacted within a reasonable time, for (1) the administration of any treatment deemed necessary for my/our children by Dr. _____, or any of his/her associates, the preferred physician, or Dr. _____, or any of his/her associates, the preferred dentist, or in the event the appropriate preferred practitioner is not available, by another licensed, qualified physician or dentist; and (2) the transfer of any of my/our children to _____ Hospital, the preferred hospital, or any hospital reasonably accessible.

MAJOR SURGERY

This authorization does not cover nonemergency major surgery unless the medical opinions of two other licensed physicians or dentists concurring in the necessity for such surgery are obtained prior to the performance of such surgery and unless all reasonable attempts to contact me/us have been unsuccessful, defining such period for nonemergency surgery as 24 hours.

MEDICAL DATA

The following is needed by any hospital or practitioner not having access to my/our children's medical history:

Allergies: _____

Medication being taken: _____

Physical impairments: _____

Other pertinent facts to which physician should be alerted: _____

Medical insurance coverage: _____

I/we, the undersigned parent(s), also do by these premises appoint and constitute _____ and _____ and/or _____ as temporary custodians of my/our children above mentioned, for the period of _____, 20 ____, through and including _____, 20 ____, and do hereby authorize them to obtain any X-ray examination, anesthesia, medical or surgical diagnosis or treatment, and hospital care to be rendered to my/our children in our absence, under the general or special supervision, and on the advice of, a licensed physician, surgeon, anesthesiologist, dentist, or other qualified personnel acting under their supervision.

Witnesses _____

_____

State of _____

SS: _____

_____ County

Note: The law varies from state to state. No form should be adopted or used by any program without individualized legal advice.

Reprinted, by permission, from D. Herbert, 1994, *Legal aspects of sports medicine*, 2nd ed. (Canton, OH: Professional Reports Corporation).

Form 15

Fitness Evaluation Form

Date _____ / _____ / _____

Member name _____ Membership number _____

Member address _____ City _____ State _____ (Zip) _____ Member phone number _____

Physician's name _____

Physician's address _____ City _____ State _____ (Zip) _____ Physician's phone number _____

I. General physiological information   Birth date _____ / _____ / _____
1. Age _____   2. Sex M ☐ F ☐ 3. Risk category _____   4. Height _____ ft _____ in.
5. Weight _____ 6. RHR _____ 7. RBP _____   8. Predicted Max HR _____
Medications_____   _____
Exercise history _____

II. Cardiovascular assessment
1. RHR supine_____
2. RBP supine _____
3. RBP standing_____
4. Predicted heart rate

Max _____
90% _____
80% _____
70% _____

5. HVHR _____
Protocol _____
Equipment _____
Max HR _____ Max BP ____/____
Max met _____

Stage	Time	Speed KPM	Grade	HR	BP	DP	ST	Comments
1	1							
	2							
	3							
2	1							
	2							
	3							
3	1							
	2							
	3							
4	1							
	2							
	3							
5	1							
	2							
	3							
R e s t	1							
	3							
	6							
	9							

III. Lung capacity
1. Vital capacity ___/___% Pred.
2. FEV   ___/___% Pred.

IV. Flexibility
1. Sit'n'reach ___ ___ ___in.

V. Muscular strength and endurance
1. Grip ___/___/___ KgR ___/___/___KgL
2. Trunk curl/sit-up _____#_____ Time
3. _____   _____

VI. Body composition

A. Skin folds   1   2   Avg.
1. Chest   _____ _____ _____
2. Subscapula   _____ _____ _____
3. Suprailliac _____ _____ _____
4. Umbilical   _____ _____ _____
5. Tricep   _____ _____ _____
6. Ant. thigh   _____ _____ _____
Total skin folds   _____

B. Body fat
1. Percent fat _____ %
2. Fat wt. _____ lb
3. Lean wt. _____ lb
4. Ideal percent fat ___ %
5. Ideal wt. _____ lb

C. Girths
1. Neck   _____
2. Shoulder   _____
3. Chest   _____
4. Waist   _____
5. Hips   _____
6. Thigh   ___ R ___ L
7. Calf   ___ R ___ L
8. Bicep   ___ R ___ L
9. Forearm ___ R ___ L

VII. Blood chemistry
1. Cholesterol _____
2. Chol./HDL _____
3. LDL/HDL _____
4. Triglycerides _____
5. Glucose _____
6. Hematocrit _____

Note: RHR = resting heart rate; RBP = resting blood pressure; MET = unit of metabolic measurement; HVHR = hyperventilating heart rate; FEV = forced expiratory volume; HR = heart rate; BP = blood pressure; DP = double product; ST = S-T segment; KgR = kilogram right hand; KgL = kilogram left hand. The law varies from state to state. No form should be adopted or used by any program without individualized legal advice.

Form 16

Fitness Integration Tracking Form

Member's name _____ Age ____ Acct.# _____ Acct. type ____

Consultation appt. Date/time _____ Fit specialist _____ Coach _____

REASONS	
(check)	(rank)
☐ Lose body fat	_____
☐ Stress release	_____
☐ Meet similar folk	_____
☐ Family recreation	_____
☐ Strengthen/Tone	_____
☐ Self-esteem increase	_____
☐ Energy level increase	_____
☐ _____	_____

INTERESTS		
☐ Lose body fat	☐ Karate	☐ Personal training
☐ Weight training	☐ Massage	☐ Child care
☐ Swimming	☐ Water exercise classes	☐ Physical therapy
☐ Exercise group classes	☐ Fitness evaluation	☐ Nutrition
☐ Youth activities	☐ Swim lessons	☐ Social events
☐ Racquetball	☐ Sports leagues	☐ Volleyball
☐ Basketball	☐ Fitness leagues	☐ _____
☐ Sauna/steam	☐ Jacuzzi	☐ _____

SUCCESS PLAN

1. My MAIN objective is: _____

2. Why? _____

3. How will this accomplishment make you feel? _____

4. When would you like to accomplish this? _____

5. Why by then? _____

6. Baby Steps: _____

7. Will you need support in accomplishing these steps or changes? yes/no

    From whom? (family, training coach, social group, work peers, etc.) _____

8. What days of the week do you see yourself using the Club (circle) S M T W Th F S

9. Time of day? _____ # of Club visits per week?_____

10. Are #8 and #9 above realistic for you? yes/no_____

11. If you consistently follow through on Baby Steps, how will you feel? _____

12. Do you foresee any potential obstacle or distractions? _____

13. How can I assist you in accomplishing your goals?_____

14. What type of coaching/support would benefit you most?

     _____

15. Notes: _____

     _____

Adapted, by permission, from East Side Athletic Club (Milwaukie, OR: East Side Athletic Club).

Form 17

Cardiovascular Assessment Data Sheet

Name _____ Date _____ Age _____

Weight (kg) _____ Resting heart rate _____

Age-predicted max heart rate

60% _____ 65% _____ 70% _____ 90% _____

Mode of cardiovascular evaluation: bike RPMs _____, treadmill (please circle one)

  I. Warm-up workload: _____

   1 min _____   RPE _____

   2 min _____   BP _____

   3 min _____

   4 min _____

 II. Target workload #1: _____

   1 min _____   RPE _____

   2 min _____   BP _____

   3 min _____

   4 min _____

III. Target workload #2 (if indicated): _____

   1 min _____   RPE _____

   2 min _____   BP _____

   3 min _____

   4 min _____

 IV. Cool-down workload: _____

   1 min _____   RPE _____

   2 min _____   BP _____

  V. $\dot{V}O_2$ max calculation conversion to METs:

   Predicted $\dot{V}O_2$ max (L/min) _____ × age factor _____ = maximum $\dot{V}O_2$ (L/min) _____

   $\dot{V}O_2$ max (ml/min) _____ – wt (kg) _____ = $\dot{V}O_2$ max (ml/kg/min) _____

   $\dot{V}O_2$ max (ml/kg/min) _____ – 3.5 = predicted maximal capacity in METs

 VI. Summary

   • Predicted maximal capacity (METs) _____

   • Recommended training range (METs) _____

   • Recommended training range (heart rate) _____

Note: BP = blood pressure; MET = unit of metabolic measurement; RPM = rotations per minute; RPE = rate of perceived exertion.
The law varies from state to state. No form should be adopted or used by any program without individualized legal advice.

Form 18

Release of Information Form

To whom it may concern:

Please be advised that (_____) and any member, associate, or designee of that firm is hereby authorized to inspect and copy or be furnished copies of any and all hospital, dental, or medical records of any sort as well as charts, notes, medical bills, dental bills, X-rays, lab reports, and prescriptions and is to be furnished any and all other information without limitations pertaining to any confinement, examination, treatment, or condition of myself, including medical, dental, psychological, or other treatment; examinations; or counseling for any medical, dental, or psychological condition.

This authorization shall be considered as continuing and you may rely on it in all respects unless you have previously been advised by me in writing to the contrary. It is expressly understood by the undersigned and you are hereby authorized to accept a copy or photocopy of this medical authorization with the same validity as though an original had been presented to you.

Dated this _____ day of _____, 20 _____.

X _____

Note: The law varies from state to state. No form should be adopted or used by any program without individualized legal advice.

Reprinted, by permission, from B.E. Koeberle, 1990, *Legal aspects of personal fitness training* (Canton, OH: Professional Reports Corporation), 149.

Form 19

Progress Notes

Date _____

Physician _____

Member's name _____

Weight _____ Date of last program review _____

Medical history changes _____

_____

_____

Exercise prescription _____

_____

_____

Comments _____

_____

_____

Form 20
Incident Report Form

Date of accident _____ Time of accident _____

Member's name _____ Member number _____

Address _____

Home phone _____ Business phone _____

Location of accident _____

Staff attending _____ _____

_____ _____

Witnesses (nonstaff) _____ _____

_____ _____

Details of accident _____

_____

_____

_____

Action taken by staff _____

_____

_____

_____

Staff reporting _____ Date _____

Department head's signature _____ Date _____

Note: The law varies from state to state. No form should be adopted or used by any program without individualized legal advice.

Form 21

Theft Report Form

Date of incident _____ Time of incident _____

Item reported missing _____

Member's name _____ Member number _____

Address _____

Home phone _____ Business phone _____

Location of incident _____

Description of incident _____

_____

_____

_____

Witnesses _____   _____

_____   _____

Reporting by _____ Date and time _____

Action taken _____

_____

_____

_____

Supervisor's signature _____ Date _____

Form 22

Sample Exercise Card

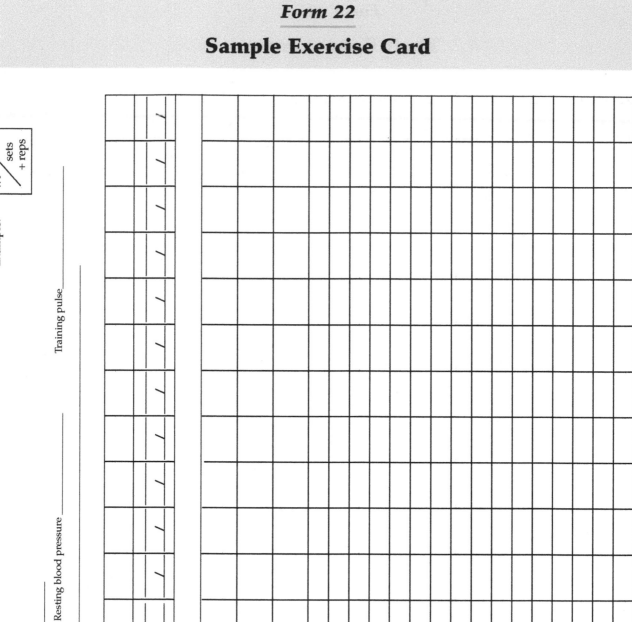

Please see your motivator when finished with your card.

Form 23

Physical Activity Readiness Medical Exam Form (PARmed-X)

The PARmed-X is a physical activity-specific checklist to be used by a physician with patients who have had positive responses to the Physical Activity Readiness Questionnaire (PAR-Q). In addition, the Conveyance/Referral Form in the PARmed-X can be used to convey clearance for physical activity participation, or to make a referral to a medically-supervised exercise program.

Regular physical activity is fun and healthy, and increasingly more people are starting to become more active every day. Being more active is very safe for most people. The PAR-Q by itself provides adequate screening for the majority of people. However, some individuals may require a medical evaluation and specific advice (exercise prescription) due to one or more positive responses to the PAR-Q.

Following the participant's evaluation by a physician, a physical activity plan should be devised in consultation with a physical activity professional (CSEP-Certified Fitness Appraiser). To assist in this, the following instructions are provided:

Page 1: • Sections A, B, C, and D should be completed by the participant BEFORE the examination by the physician. The bottom section is to be completed by the examining physician.

Pages 2 & 3: • A checklist of medical conditions requiring special consideration and management.

This section to be completed by the participant

A PERSONAL INFORMATION:

Name _____

Address _____

_____

Telephone _____

Birth date _____ Gender _____

Medical No. _____

B PAR-Q: Please indicate the PAR-Q questions to which you answered YES

☐ Q1. Heart condition
☐ Q2. Chest pain during activity
☐ Q3. Chest pain at rest
☐ Q4. Loss of balance, dizziness
☐ Q5. Bone or joint problem
☐ Q6. Blood pressure or heart drugs
☐ Q7. Other reason:

C RISK FACTORS FOR CARDIOVASCULAR DISEASE:

Check all that apply

☐ Less than 30 minutes of moderate physical activity most days of the week.
☐ Currently smoker (tobacco smoking 1 or more times per week).
☐ High blood pressure reported by physician after repeated measurements.
☐ High cholesterol level reported by physician.

☐ Excessive accumulation of fat around waist.
☐ Family history of heart disease.

Please note: Many of these risk factors are modifiable. Please discuss with your physician.

D PHYSICAL ACTIVITY INTENTIONS:

What physical activity do you intend to do?

_____

_____

_____

This section to be completed by the examining physician

Physical Exam:

Ht	Wt		BP i)	/
			BP ii)	/

Conditions limiting physical activity:

☐ Cardiovascular   ☐ Respiratory   ☐ Other
☐ Musculoskeletal   ☐ Abdominal

Tests required:

☐ ECG   ☐ Exercise test   ☐ X-Ray
☐ Blood   ☐ Urinalysis   ☐ Other

Physical Activity Readiness Conveyance/Referral:
Based upon a current review of health status, I recommend:

☐ No physical activity

☐ Only a medically-supervised exercise program until further medical clearance

☐ Progressive physical activity
  ☐ with avoidance of: _____
  ☐ with inclusion of: _____
  ☐ with Physical Therapy: _____

☐ Unrestricted physical activity —start slowly and build up gradually

Further information:
☐ Attached
☐ To be forwarded
☐ Available on request

(continued)

(continued)

Following is a checklist of medical conditions for which a degree of precaution and/or special advice should be considered for those who answered "YES" to one or more questions on the PAR-Q, and people over the age of 69. Conditions are grouped by system. Three categories of precautions are provided. Comments under Advice are general, since details and alternatives require clinical judgment in each individual instance.

	Absolute Contraindications	**Relative Contraindications**	**Special Prescriptive Conditions**	**Advice**
	Permanent restriction or temporary restriction until condition is treated, stable, and/or past acute phase.	Highly variable. Value of exercise testing and/or program may exceed risk. Activity may be restricted. Desirable to maximize control of condition. Direct or indirect medical supervision or exercise program may be desirable.	Individualized prescriptive advice generally appropriate: • limitations imposed; and/or • special exercises prescribed. May require medical monitoring and/or initial supervision in exercise program.	

Cardiovascular	❑ aortic aneurysm (dissecting)
	❑ aortic stenosis (severe)
	❑ congestive heart failure
	❑ crescendo angina
	❑ myocardial infarction (acute)
	❑ myocarditis (active or recent)
	❑ pulmonary or systemic embolism—acute
	❑ thrombophlebitis
	❑ ventricular tachycardia and other dangerous dysrhythmias (e.g., multi-focal ventricular activity)
		❑ aortic stenosis (moderate)
		❑ subaortic stenosis (severe)
		❑ marked cardiac enlargement
		❑ supraventricular dysrhythmias (uncontrolled or high rate)
		❑ ventricular ectopic activity (repetitive or frequent)
		❑ ventricular aneurysm
		❑ hypertension—untreated or uncontrolled severe (systemic or pulmonary)
		❑ hypertrophic cardiomyopathy
		❑ compensated congestive heart failure
			❑ aortic (or pulmonary) stenosis—mild angina pectoris and other manifestations of coronary insufficiency (e.g., post-acute infarct)
			❑ cyanotic heart disease
			❑ shunts (intermittent or fixed)
			❑ conduction disturbances
			  • complete AV block
			  • left BBB
			  • Wolff-Parkinson-White syndrome
			❑ dysrhythmias—controlled
			❑ fixed rate pacemakers
				• clinical exercise test may be warranted in selected cases, for specific determination of functional capacity and limitations and precautions (if any).
				• slow progression of exercise to levels based on test performance and individual tolerance.
				• consider individual need for initial conditioning program under medical supervision (indirect or direct).

			❑ intermittent claudication	progressive exercise to tolerance
			❑ hypertension: systolic 160-180; diastolic 105+	progressive exercise; care with medications (serum electrolytes; post-exercise syncope; etc.)
Infections	❑ acute infectious disease (regardless of etiology)	❑ subacute/chronic/recurrent infectious diseases (e.g., malaria, others)	❑ chronic infections ❑ HIV	variable as to condition
Metaboli		❑ uncontrolled metabolic disorders (diabetes mellitus, thyrotoxicosis, myxedema)	❑ renal, hepatic, & other metabolic insufficiency	variable as to status
			❑ obesity ❑ single kidney	dietary moderation, and initial light exercises with slow progression (walking, swimming, cycling)
Pregnancy		❑ complicated pregnancy (e.g., toxemia, hemorrhage, incompetent cervix, etc.)	❑ advanced pregnancy (late 3rd trimester)	refer to the "PARmed-X for PREGNANCY"

References:

Arraix, G.A., Wigle, D.T., Mao, Y. (1992). Risk Assessment of Physical Activity and Physical Fitness in the Canada Health Survey Follow-Up Study. **J. Clin. Epidemiol. 45:4 419-428.**

Mottola, M., Wolfe, L.A. (1994). Active Living and Pregnancy, In: A. Quinney, L. Gauvin, T. Wall (eds), **Toward Active Living: Proceedings of the International Conference on Physical Activity, Fitness, and Health.** Champaign, IL: Human Kinetics.

PAR-Q Validation Report, British Columbia Ministry of Health, 1978.

Thomas, S., Reading, J., Shephard, R.J. (1992). Revision of the Physical Activity Readiness Questionnaire (PAR-Q). **Can. J. Spt. Sci.** 17:4 338-345.

	Special Prescriptive Conditions	Advice
Lung	❏ chronic pulmonary disorders	special relaxation and breathing exercises
	❏ obstructive lung disease ❏ asthma	breath control during endurance exercise to tolerance; avoid polluted air
	❏ exercise-induced bronchospasm	avoid hyperventilation during exercise; avoid extremely cold conditions; warm up adequately; utilize appropriate medication
Musculoskeletal	❏ low back conditions (pathological, functional)	avoid or minimize exercise that precipitates or exacerbates (e.g., forced extreme flexion, extension, and violent twisting); correct posture, proper back exercises
	❏ arthritis—acute (infective, rheumatoid; gout)	treatment, plus judicious blend of rest, splinting, and gentle movement
	❏ arthritis—subacute	progressive increase of active exercise therapy
	❏ arthritis—chronic (osteoarthritis and above conditions)	maintenance of mobility and strength; non-weightbearing exercises to minimize joint trauma (e.g., cycling, aquatic activity, etc.)
	❏ orthopaedic	highly variable and individualized
	❏ hernia	minimize straining and isometrics; strengthen abdominal muscles
CNS	❏ convulsive disorder not completely controlled by medication	minimize or avoid exercise in hazardous environments and/or exercising alone (e.g., swimming, mountain climbing, etc.)
	❏ recent concussion	thorough examination if history of two concussions; review for discontinuation of contact sport if three concussions, depending on duration of unconsciousness, retrograde amnesia, persistent headaches, and other objective evidence of cerebral damage
Blood	❏ anemia—severe (< 10 Gm/dl) ❏ electrolyte disturbances	control preferred; exercise as tolerated
Medications	❏ antianginal ❏ antiarrhythmic ❏ antihypertensive ❏ anticonvulsant ❏ beta-blockers ❏ digitalis preparations ❏ diuretics ❏ ganglionic blockers ❏ others	NOTE: consider underlying condition. Potential for: exertional syncope, electrolyte imbalance, bradycardia, dysrhythmias, impaired coordinations and reaction time, heat intolerance. May alter resting and exercise ECG's and exercise test performance.
Other	❏ post-exercise syncope	moderate program
	❏ heat intolerance	prolong cool-down with light activities; avoid exercise in extreme heat
	❏ temporary minor illness	postpone until recovered
	❏ cancer	if potential metastases, test by cycle ergometry, consider non-weight bearing exercises; exercise at lower end of prescriptive range (40-65% of heart rate reserve), depending on condition and recent treatment (radiation, chemotherapy); monitor hemoglobin and lymphocyte counts; add dynamic lifting exercises to strengthen muscles, using machines rather than weights.

* Refer to special publications for elaboration as required.

Form 24

Emergency Procedures Sheet

In the event that an emergency should occur and no medical personnel are present, the following guidelines should be followed:

1. A staff person should identify him or herself as a professional rescuer trained in emergency care. This helps to reassure the victim and bystanders. If the victim is conscious, legally we must ask permission to assist the victim. (The law assumes that an unconscious person would give consent.) A senior staff person should stay with the individual at all times. He or she should attempt to reassure the person and protect the individual from personal bodily harm. Senior staff person will assume control of the situation and issue further orders as needed.

2. A second staff member will call 911 and give the following information:
   A. Phone number of location
   B. Title of location (building name, address, specific suite or room number)
   C. Site-specific entrance instructions for ambulance driver
   D. Brief description of the problem. If it is a definite cardiac event (i.e., respiratory arrest) and CPR is in progress, an Advanced Life Support unit will be sent. If it is nonlife-threatening (i.e., seizures), a Basic Life Support unit will be sent.
   E. After 911 has been called, a staff member will notify building security (list phone #: _____), put elevator on hold (if applicable), and wait in the lobby to meet the ambulance at the main entrance to escort them to the emergency.

3. The individual should be monitored at all times. This will include:
   A. Checking heart rate, noting the regularity and strength of each heart beat.
   B. Monitoring and recording blood pressure.
   C. Observing skin color and breathing pattern.
   D. Maintaining open airway.
   E. Establishing unresponsiveness and initiating CPR when appropriate.
   F. Before the individual is transported (if unconscious), give the EMTs as much information as possible regarding individual's name, age, medical considerations (folder, if possible), and home phone emergency numbers. The attending physician and the hospital will make the call to the family.

4. Once the individual is transported, the senior staff person in charge should:
   A. Notify the individual's work place so that the employer can decide how to handle the family.
   B. Assume responsibility for personal belongings and valuables. Please remember that it is important to respect the individual's privacy. Be as brief as possible when disclosing the information pertinent to the event.
   C. Fill out an accident report and file one copy in the member's folder and one copy with the Center Director.

Form 25

Health Questionnaire

Name _____ Date _____

Address _____

Gender _____ Birthday _____ E-mail _____

Telephone (W) _____ Telephone (H) _____

Regular physical activity is fun and healthy and for most people safe. However, some individuals may have health-related risks that might require them to check with their physician prior to starting an exercise program. To help determine if there is a need for you to see your physician before starting an exercise program, please read the following questions and answer carefully.

All information will be kept in the strictest confidentiality. In addition to the health history questions, we have also listed several questions pertaining to your interests and goals for participating in an exercise/physical activity program.

I. PHYSICAL ACTIVITY SCREENING QUESTIONS

Yes *No*

☐ ☐   1. Has your physician ever told you that you have a heart condition?
☐ ☐   2. Do you experience pain in your chest when you are physically active?
☐ ☐   3. In the past month, have you experienced chest pain when not performing physical activity?
☐ ☐   4. Do you lose balance because of dizziness or do you ever lose consciousness?
☐ ☐   5. Do you have a bone or joint problem that could be aggravated by a change in your level of physical activity?
☐ ☐   6. Is your physician currently prescribing medications for your blood pressure or heart condition?
☐ ☐   7. Do you know of any other reason why you should not participate in a program of physical activity?

If you answered yes to any of the above questions, it is recommended that you consult with your physician via phone or in person before having a fitness test or participating in a physical activity program.

II. GENERAL HEALTH HISTORY QUESTIONS

Yes *No*

☐ ☐   1. Have you ever experienced a stroke?
☐ ☐   2. Do you have diabetes? If yes, are you currently taking any medications or receiving other treatment related to the diabetes? _____
☐ ☐   3. Do you have asthma or another respiratory condition that causes difficulty with breathing? If yes, please describe. _____
☐ ☐   4. Do you have any orthopedic conditions that would restrict you in performing physical activity? If yes, please describe. _____
☐ ☐   5. Have you ever been told by a physician that you have one of the following? (check applicable boxes) ☐ High blood pressure ☐ Elevated blood lipids, including cholesterol
☐ ☐   6. Do you currently smoke?
☐ ☐   7. Have you experienced within the past 6 months back pain or discomfort that prevented you from carrying out normal daily activities?
☐ ☐   8. Are you pregnant?
☐ ☐   9. Do you currently exercise less than one hour per week? If you answered no, please describe your activities: _____
☐ ☐ 10. Are you currently taking any medications that might impact your ability to safely perform physical activity?

(continued)

(continued)

I. ACTIVITY RELEASE AGREEMENT: ADULT

I am voluntarily participating in an athletic or physical activity at ("the club") with full knowledge and understanding and appreciation of the risks of injury inherent in any physical exercise, massage or therapy program, physical activity, or athletic activity and expressly assume all risks of injury and even death, which could occur by reason of my participation. I release the club from any liability and agree not to sue the club with respect to any cause of action for bodily injury, property damage, or death occurring to me as a result of my participation in the activity.

I understand that all personal property brought to the club is brought at my sole risk as to its theft, damage, or loss.

Participant   Witness
Signature _____   Signature _____

Date _____   Date _____

Printed name _____   Printed name _____

II. FOR MEMBERSHIP/ATHLETIC USE ONLY

Category 1 _____ Category 2 _____ Category 3 _____

Form 26

Coronary Risk Factor Identification Form

Member name _____ Member # _____ Date _____

Place a check next to any lines below that apply to the member.

1. _____ **Age:** (Circle)   Men >45   Women >55

2. _____ **Family history:** MI or sudden death before 55 years of age for father or other first degree male relative

    MI or sudden death before 65 years of age for mother or other first degree female relative

3. _____ **Cigarette smoker:** (Current)

4. _____ **Hypercholesterolemia:** Blood cholesterol > 200 mg/dl

5. _____ **Hypertension:** Blood pressure > 140/90 mm Hg or on hypertensive meds.

6. _____ **Diabetes mellitus:** Classified with disease as follows:
    ☐ NIDDM > 35 years or older.
    ☐ IDDM > older than 30 or having IDDM for 15 years minimum.

7. _____ **Sedentary lifestyle:** Physical inactivity.

_____ **Apparently healthy:**
Asymptomatic and apparently healthy with no more than one major coronary risk factor.

Risk factors: _____

_____

_____

_____ **Increased risk:**
An individual who has signs or symptoms suggestive of possible cardiopulmonary or metabolic disease and/or two or more major coronary risk factors.

Risk factors: _____

_____

_____

Physician's note required Date contacted: _____

_____ **Known disease:**
An individual with known cardiac, pulmonary, or metabolic disease.

Risk factors: _____

_____

_____

Physician's note required Date contacted: _____

Form 27

Fitness Testing Form

Name _____ Member # _____ Gender _____ Age _____

		INITIAL	30 DAY	60 DAY
DATE				
RESTING HR				
Resting BP				
	Systolic			
	Diastolic			
Circumferences				
	Biceps			
	Chest			
	Waist			
	Hip			
	Thigh			
Skinfolds				
	Pectoral (M)			
	Abdominal (M)			
	Thigh (F/M)			
	Tricep (F)			
	Suprailliac			
	Sum			
	% body fat			
3-minute step test				
	HR			
	Fitness level			
Push-ups				
Flexibility				
	Sit and reach			
Height				
Weight				

Form 28

Medical Clearance Form

Information requested for _____

Physician's name _____

Telephone number _____

Please sign the statement that reflects your wishes:

1. _____ I concur with my patient's participation if he/she restricts activities to those that are moderate.

2. _____ I do not concur with my patient's participation in this program. (If checked, the individual will not be accepted.)

3. _____ Other: _____

_____

Return form to: _____

Form 29

Exercise Contract

Member name _____

Member contact no. (W) _____ (H) _____ (C) _____

Fitness motivator _____

Motivator contact no. (W) _____ (H) _____ (C) _____

Goals and Objectives

My main exercise goal is to _____

To achieve my main goal, I need to do the following:

a. 30-day goal _____

_____

b. 60-day goal _____

_____

c. 90-day goal _____

_____

d. 6-month goal _____

_____

I commit to do the following:

1. Cardiovascular _____

_____

2. Strength training _____

_____

3. Nutrition _____

_____

4. Flexibility _____

_____

What barriers do you expect might arise to prevent you from achieving your goals and how can we assist in overcoming them?

Exercise Contract Overview

1. When establishing this contract with a Member, be certain to set SMART goals *(Specific, Measurable, Achievable, Realistic, and Timed)*.

2. To help achieve the desired results, use the following options as incentives to keep the Member motivated:

    a. If not yet committed to an exercise program. Additional training sessions; setting them up with an exercise "buddy" in the same exercise situation; discounts for club services such as massage, lessons, classes, etc.; educational materials on benefits of exercise; group training sessions; and incentives or rewards.

    b. If already participating in a program but just recently started. The focus is on preventing lapses (short breaks from exercise) and relapses (long periods of inactivity). Use buddy programs and group training options for social support. Additional complimentary training and incentives rewards work well also.

3. The support you provide as the motivator is critical to the success.

Form 30

Health, Fitness, and Racquet Sports Club Incident Report

(Complete for all incidents and report immediately—please print)

D A T E	Month Day Year Time of Accident A.M. P.M.	Club member ☐ Yes ☐ No	Club name Club location

I N J U R E D P E R S O N		Hospital or first aid squad notified ☐ Yes ☐ No
	First name (M.I.) Last name Age	Name:
		Time of initial call:
		Times of follow-up calls: 1. 3. 2. 4.
	Number and street	
		Time of arrival:
	City State Zip	Time of departure:
		Taken to hospital?
	Business phone	Name of first aid attendant:
	Home phone	

DESCRIPTION OF ACCIDENT:

CHECK ITEMS THAT APPLY TO INJURED PERSON:

Bleeding injury: ☐ Yes ☐ No   Other visible injury: ☐ Yes ☐ No

No visible injury, but complaint of pain: ☐ Yes ☐ No

If eye injury, wearing eyeguards? ☐ Yes ☐ No

DESCRIBE EXACT INJURY SUSTAINED:	**DESCRIBE FIRST AID ADMINISTERED BY CLUB:**

FIRST WITNESS	**SECOND WITNESS**
First name (M.I.) Last name	First name (M.I.) Last name
Number and street	Number and street
City State Zip	City State Zip
Business phone Home phone	Business phone Home phone
DESCRIPTION OF ACCIDENT BY WITNESS	**DESCRIPTION OF ACCIDENT BY WITNESS**
Signature:	Signature:

HEALTH, FITNESS & RACQUET SPORTS CLUB INCIDENT REPORT
[continued]

Name of club personnel who inspected the scene:	Position	Date of inspection

Conditions found: _____

_____

_____

_____

Action taken, if practical, to avoid recurrence: _____

_____

DESCRIPTION OF PLACE OF ACCIDENT

☐ Interior ☐ Exterior ☐ Walking area ☐ Playing surface ☐ Locker room

☐ Physical fitness room ☐ Other: _____

Conditions: ☐ Dry ☐ Wet ☐ Smooth ☐ Even surface ☐ Slippery

Foreign substance? ☐ Yes ☐ No   If "YES", description: _____

_____

If injury took place outside club building, check appropriate items:

Weather condition: ☐ Dry ☐ Rain ☐ Snow ☐ Ice ☐ Day ☐ Night   Lighting conditions: _____

IMPORTANT: If injury took place on a court, provide name, address, and telephone number of those individuals who used or rented the court during the prior hour.

_____

_____

_____

ADDITIONAL COMMENTS

_____

_____

Did police investigate?	Name and rank of officer:	Department:	Phone number
☐ Yes ☐ No			

Submitted by (signature):	Telephone:	Date / Time

This information is for reporting purposes only. The information provided is the responsibility of the insured and/or club.

Form 31
Housekeeping Checklist—Fitness Equipment Room

Note: Follow manufacturer's recommendation for maintaining belts, rods, bearings, chains, gears, and upholstered surfaces of exercise equipment.

DAILY

_____ Remove trash for disposal and replace liners

_____ Dust all horizontal surfaces

_____ Spot-clean mirrors and glass

_____ Spot-clean doors, door handles, light switches, trash containers, etc.

_____ Spot-clean walls

_____ Clean and disinfect all benches and equipment

_____ Polish vinyl pad surfaces with furniture polish

_____ Vacuum carpets

_____ Remove spots and stains from carpet

_____ Spray odor counteractant

BIMONTHLY

_____ Completely clean mirrors, rubber floor, equipment, benches, etc.

_____ Clean HVAC vents

_____ Clean light fixtures

_____ Move all equipment and clean underneath

QUARTERLY

_____ Bonnet-clean carpets

YEARLY

_____ Extraction-clean carpets

_____ Wash all walls

MAINTENANCE
Report any repairs required

_____

_____

_____

_____

_____

PEST CONTROL
Report any evidence of insects or rodents

_____

_____

_____

_____

_____

1. DAILY MAINTENANCE

A. Trash removal

Purpose: Provide a clean, well-maintained area for all members using the facility

Frequency: Daily or more frequently depending on the amount of traffic

Techniques: Remove trash and replace liners

B. Cleaning and disinfecting of workout equipment room surfaces

Purpose: Provide clean, sanitary, odor-free area for all members

Frequency: Daily or more frequently depending on the amount of traffic and soil levels

Techniques: Vacuum carpet, remove carpet spots and stains, clean and disinfect benches and equipment, spot-clean any mirror surfaces, door handles, doors, light switches, and walls

2. BIMONTHLY MAINTENANCE: FULL WET CLEANING OF ALL SURFACES

Purpose: To completely clean all room surfaces including mirrors, vents, light fixtures, rubber floor, equipment, benches, doors, etc.

Frequency: Every two weeks

Technique: Completely clean any mirrors, vents, light fixtures, rubber floor, equipment, benches, doors, etc.

3. BIMONTHLY MAINTENANCE: MOVE ALL EQUIPMENT AND CLEAN UNDERNEATH

Purpose: To completely clean all room surfaces

Frequency: Every two weeks

Technique: Move all equipment and clean underneath, vacuum or dust mop and damp mop as required

4. QUARTERLY MAINTENANCE: CARPET CLEANING

Purpose: To clean traffic lanes of carpet and maintain a high level of appearance

Frequency: Every three months

Technique: Bonnet-clean carpets

5. YEARLY MAINTENANCE: CARPET CLEANING AND WALL WASHING

Purpose: Provide a high level of appearance and odor free environment

Frequency: Yearly

Technique: Clean carpets and wash walls

Courtesy of Ecolab.

Form 32

Housekeeping Checklist—Locker Room

Date _____

Housekeeper _____

DAILY

_____ Remove trash for disposal and replace liners

_____ Refill paper, hand soap, shampoo, conditioner dispensers, etc.

_____ Dust and polish all furniture and touch-up other wood surfaces

_____ Dust all horizontal surfaces

_____ Spot-clean mirrors and glass

_____ Spot-clean doors, door handles, light switches, trash containers, etc.

_____ Spot-clean walls

_____ Spot-clean lockers

_____ Clean and disinfect sinks, commodes, urinals, etc.

_____ Clean and disinfect showers, sauna, steam room, and whirlpool

_____ Vacuum carpets

_____ Remove spots and stains from carpet

_____ Dust mop or sweep hard surface floors

_____ Wet mop and disinfect hard surface floors

_____ Spray odor counteractant

BIMONTHLY

_____ Clean mirrors, glass, and locker surfaces completely

_____ Clean hard surface floors by scrubbing with deck brush or machine

_____ Clean and disinfect showers, steam room, sauna, and whirlpool

_____ Clean HVAC vents

_____ Clean light fixtures

MONTHLY

_____ Refill air freshener dispensers

QUARTERLY

_____ Bonnet-clean carpets

YEARLY

_____ Extraction-clean carpets

_____ Wash all walls

MAINTENANCE
Report any repairs required

_____

_____

_____

_____

PEST CONTROL
Report any evidence of insects or rodents

_____

_____

_____

_____

OVERVIEW

1. **Daily Maintenance**

   A. **Trash removal, refilling paper supplies and hand soap and other dispensers**

   Purpose: Provide a well-maintained locker room for all members using the facility

   Frequency: Daily or more frequently depending on the amount of traffic

   Techniques: Refill all toilet paper, paper towel, seat covers, and liquid hand soap dispensers

   B. **Cleaning and disinfecting of locker room surfaces**

   Purpose: Provide clean, sanitary, odor-free locker room area for all members

   Frequency: Daily or more frequently depending on the amount of traffic and soil levels

   Techniques: Wet cleaning and disinfecting of all surfaces, including lockers, fixtures, showers, walls, partitions, steam room, sauna, whirlpool, floors, and wood surface touch-up

   Spot mop cleaning and disinfecting should be performed on spills when they occur

2. **Bimonthly Maintenance: Full Wet Cleaning and Disinfecting**

   Purpose: To completely clean and disinfect all locker room surfaces including lockers, fixtures, showers, walls, partitions, steam room, sauna, whirlpool, and doors; clean and polish furniture and other wood surfaces

   Frequency: Every two weeks

   Technique: Completely clean and disinfect fixtures, walls, floors, vents, and light fixtures

3. **Quarterly Maintenance: Carpet Cleaning**

   Purpose: To clean traffic lanes of carpet and maintain a high level of appearance

   Frequency: Every three months

   Technique: Bonnet-clean carpets

4. **Yearly Maintenance: Carpet Extraction Cleaning and Wall Washing**

   Purpose: Provide a high level of appearance and odor free environment

   Frequency: Yearly

   Technique: Extraction-clean carpets and wash walls

Accessible Sports Facilities

A Summary of Accessibility Guidelines for Recreational Facilities

INTRODUCTION

The Americans with Disabilities Act (ADA) is a comprehensive civil rights law that prohibits discrimination on the basis of disability. The ADA requires that newly constructed and altered state and local government facilities, places of public accommodation, and commercial facilities be readily accessible to, and usable by, individuals with disabilities. The ADA Accessibility Guidelines (ADAAG) is the standard applied to buildings and facilities. Recreational facilities, including sports facilities, are among the facilities required to comply with the ADA.

The Access Board issued accessibility guidelines for newly constructed and altered recreation facilities in 2002. The recreation facility guidelines are a supplement to ADAAG. As a supplement, they must be used in conjunction with ADAAG. References to ADAAG are mentioned throughout this summary. Copies of ADAAG and the recreation facility accessibility guidelines can be obtained through the Board's website at www.access-board. gov or by calling 1-800-872-2253 or 1-800-993-2822 (TTY). Once these guidelines are adopted by the Department of Justice (DOJ), all newly designed, constructed, and altered recreation facilities covered by the ADA will be required to comply.

The recreation facility guidelines cover the following facilities and elements:

- Amusement rides
- Boating facilities
- Bowling lanes
- Exercise equipment
- Fishing piers and platforms
- Golf courses
- Miniature golf courses
- Shooting facilities
- Swimming pools, wading pools, and spas

This guide is intended to help designers and operators in using the accessibility guidelines for sports facilities. These guidelines establish minimum accessibility requirements for newly designed or newly constructed and altered sports facilities. This guide is not a collection of sports facility designs. Rather, it provides specifications for elements within a sports facility to create a general level of usability for individuals with disabilities. Emphasis is placed on ensuring that individuals with disabilities are generally able to access the sports facility and use a variety of elements.

Designers and operators are encouraged to exceed the guidelines where possible to provide increased accessibility and opportunities. Incorporating accessibility into the design of a sports facility should begin early in the planning process with careful consideration of accessible routes.

The recreation facility guidelines were developed with significant public participation. In 1993, the Access Board established an advisory committee of 27 members to recommend accessibility guidelines for recreation facilities. The Recreation Access Advisory Committee represented the following groups and associations:

- American Ski Federation
- American Society for Testing and Materials (Public Playground Safety Committee)
- American Society of Landscape Architects
- Beneficial Designs
- City and County of San Francisco, California, Department of Public Works
- Disabled American Veterans
- Environmental Access
- Gold Course Superintendents Association of America
- Hawaii Disability and Communication Access Board
- International Association of Amusement Parks and Attractions
- Katherine McGuinness and Associates
- Lehman, Smith, and Wiseman Associates
- Michigan Department of Natural Resources
- National Council on Independent Living
- National Park Service
- National Recreation and Park Association
- New Jersey Department of Community Affairs
- Outdoor Amusement Business Association
- Paralyzed Veterans of America
- Professional Golfer's Association
- Self Help for Hard of Hearing People
- States Organization for Boating Access
- Universal Studios
- U.S. Army Corps of Engineers
- U.S. Forest Service
- YMCA of the USA
- Walt Disney Imagineering

The public was given an opportunity to comment on the recommended accessibility guidelines, and the Access Board made changes to the recommended guidelines based on the public comments. A notice of proposed rulemaking (NPRM) was published in the Federal Register in July 1999, followed by a five-month public comment period. Further input from the public was sought in July 2000 when the Access Board published a draft final rule soliciting comment. A final rule was published in September 2002.

"Whenever a door is closed to anyone because of a disability, we must work to open it. . . . Whenever any barrier stands between you and the full rights and dignity of citizenship, we must work to remove it, in the name of simple decency and justice. The promise of the ADA . . . has enabled people with disabilities to enjoy much greater access to a wide range of affordable travel, recreational opportunities, and life-enriching services."

—*President George W. Bush,*
New Freedom Initiative,
February 1, 2001

SPORTS FACILITIES

The recreation facility guidelines described in this guide focus on the accessible features of unique sports-related elements in newly designed or newly constructed and altered facilities. Other provisions contained in ADAAG address elements commonly found within a sports facility, such as accessible vehicle parking spaces, exterior accessible routes, doors, assembly sections, and toilet and bathing facilities. ADAAG addresses only the built environment (structures and grounds). The guidelines do not address operational issues. Questions regarding operational issues should be directed to the Department of Justice, 1-800-514-0301 or 1-800-514-0383 (TTY).

Facilities and elements covered include:

- Areas of indoor and outdoor sports activity, including court sports (such as tennis, volleyball, and racquetball), field sports (such as softball, football, lacrosse, baseball, and soccer), and other sports (such as gymnastics and wrestling)
- Dressing, fitting, and locker rooms
- Team or player seating areas
- Exercise equipment and machines

- Saunas and steam rooms
- Animal containment areas for public use such as petting zoos and passageways along animal pens at fairs
- Bowling lanes
- Shooting facilities

These recreation facility guidelines do not apply to:

- Raised structures used for refereeing, judging, or scoring a sport
- Animal containment areas not for public use
- Raised boxing rings and wrestling rings
- Water slides (as long as an accessible route is provided to the base)

ACCESSIBLE ROUTES

Accessible routes are continuous, unobstructed paths connecting all accessible elements and spaces of a building or facility. The accessible route must comply with ADAAG provisions for the location, width (minimum of 36 inches), passing space, head room, surface, slope (maximum of 1:12 or 8.33

percent), changes in level, doors, egress, and areas of rescue assistance, unless otherwise modified by specific provisions outlined in this guide. Facilities must provide accessible routes connecting all accessible elements and spaces within areas of indoor or outdoor sports activities. If not all elements need to be accessible, only those that are accessible must be connected with an accessible route.

The guidelines apply to "fixed" facilities and elements. They do not cover equipment that is frequently moved. For example, a wrestling mat or badminton net may be portable and moved regularly.

Court Sports

Where courts are provided, an accessible route must connect each court. Accessible routes must comply with all ADAAG requirements, such as width and changes in level or surface, and must directly connect both sides of the court. Players must not be required to traverse through another court to get to the other side of their court. This is especially critical in sports like tennis, in which changing sides of the court is part of the game. No additional accessibility guidelines apply once on the court.

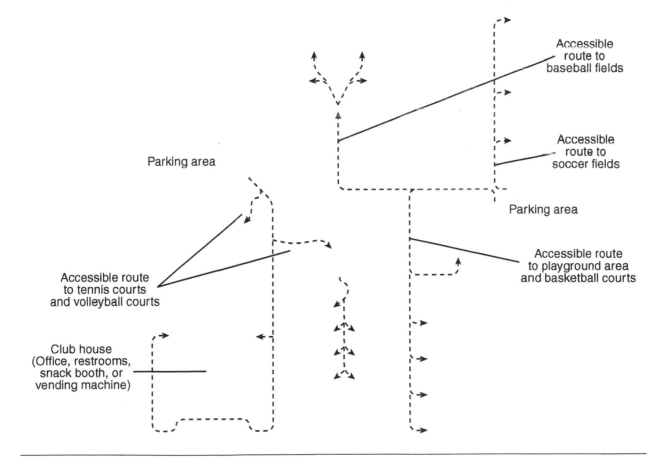

Accessible route connecting various elements of a multiuse facility.

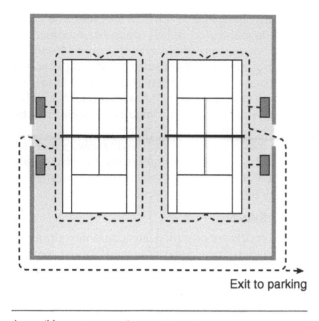

Exit to parking

Accessible route connecting court sports.

Areas of Sport Activities

An "area of sport activity" is a broad term intended to cover a diverse number of indoor and outdoor sports fields and areas. This includes, but is not limited to: basketball courts, baseball fields, running tracks, soccer fields, and skating rinks.

The "area of sport activity" is "that portion of a room or space where the play or practice of a sport occurs." For example, football fields are defined by boundary lines. In addition, a safety border is provided around the field. Players may temporarily be in the space between the boundary lines and the safety border when they are pushed out of bounds or momentum carries them forward when receiving a pass. So in football, that space is used as part of the game and is included in the area of sport activity.

Accessible routes must connect each area of sport activity. Areas of sport activities must comply with all ADAAG requirements, except that they are exempt from the requirement that surfaces must be stable, firm, and slip resistant, and from the restrictions on carpets, grating, and changes in level. They are also exempt from restrictions on protruding objects. These provisions are not required inside of the area of sport activity since they may affect the fundamental nature of the sport or activity. For example, an accessible route is required to connect to the boundary of a soccer field, but there is no requirement to change the surface of a field to an accessible surface.

Where light fixtures or gates are provided as part of a court sport or other area of sport activity, they must comply with ADAAG provisions for controls and operating mechanisms, and for gates and doors.

Animal Containment Areas

If the public has access to an animal containment area, accessible routes must connect to each animal containment area. Examples may include petting zoos, petting farms, public pathways for viewing livestock display tents, or other areas where the public has access to animals. These areas must comply with all ADAAG requirements, except the requirements that surfaces be stable, firm, and slip resistant and the restrictions on changes in level since some surfaces need to be absorbent. Accessibility is not required in areas that are for animal handlers and not for public use.

DRESSING, FITTING, OR LOCKER ROOMS

When provided, dressing, fitting, or locker rooms must be accessible and comply with all ADAAG provisions. If they are in a cluster, 5 percent, or at least one, must be accessible. There must be an accessible route through the door and to all elements required to be accessible in the room. Operating mechanisms provided on accessible lockers must also meet ADAAG provisions for their operation and height.

LOCKERS

If lockers are provided, at least 5 percent, but not less than one of each type (full, half, quarter, etc.), must be accessible. Accessible benches should be located adjacent to the accessible lockers.

BENCHES

Accessible benches are required in dressing, fitting, and locker rooms, and where seating is provided in saunas and steam rooms. Benches must have a clear floor space positioned to allow persons using wheelchairs or other mobility devices to approach parallel to the short end of a bench seat. In saunas and steam rooms, this floor space may be obstructed by readily removable seats.

Benches must have seats that are a minimum of 20 inches to a maximum of 24 inches in depth and 42 inches minimum in length. The seat height should be a minimum of 17 inches to a maximum

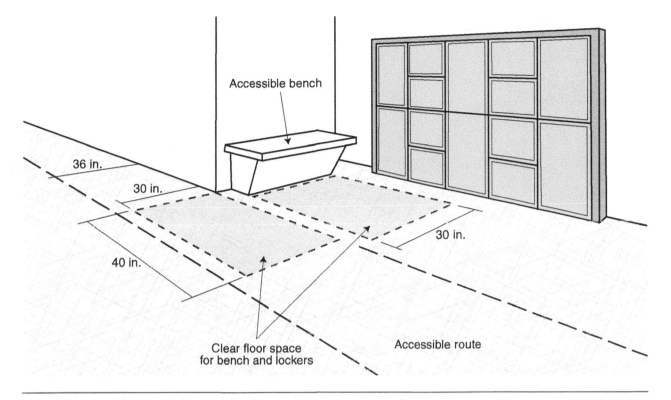

Accessible lockers.

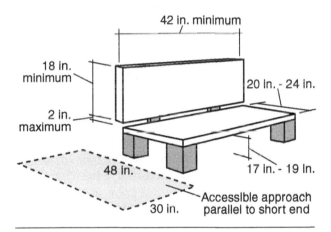

Accessible bench.

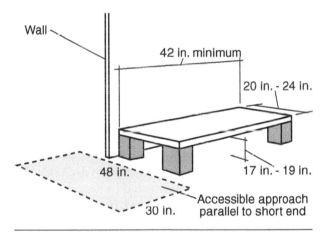

Accessible bench against a wall.

of 19 inches above the finished floor. If the bench is not located next to a wall, the bench must have back support that is 42 inches minimum in length and extends from a point 2 inches maximum above the seat to a point 18 inches minimum above the bench. Benches must be strong enough to withstand a vertical or horizontal force of 250 pounds applied at any point on the seat, fastener, mounting device, or supporting structure. The provisions for benches are not intended to apply to park benches or other benches used for sitting or resting.

If benches are located in wet areas, the surface must be slip-resistant and designed not to accumulate water.

TEAM PLAYER SEATING AREAS

Where provided, fixed team or player seating areas must contain the number of wheelchair spaces and companion seats required by ADAAG (based on the number of seats provided), but not less than one space. One option is to provide a clear space

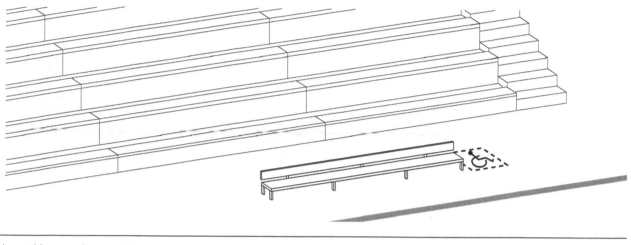

Accessible team player seating area.

adjacent to a fixed bench, with the bench serving as companion seating. If designers and operators are designing a field or court that will serve a variety of wheelchair sports, exceeding the minimum requirements will better accommodate participants.

Wheelchair spaces in the team player seating areas are exempt from the requirements related to admission price and line of sight choices in assembly areas. It is recommended that ramps be used wherever possible for accessible routes connecting team or player seating areas and areas of sport activity. However, a platform lift may be used as part of an accessible route to team player seating areas.

SAUNAS AND STEAM ROOMS

If saunas or steam rooms are in a cluster, at least 5 percent, but not less than one of each type, must be accessible. The wheelchair turning space in the sauna or steam room must comply with ADAAG, except that it can be obstructed by readily removable seats. If seating is provided, at least one bench must be accessible. Doors cannot swing into any part of the clear floor or ground space required for benches.

EXERCISE EQUIPMENT AND MACHINES

At least one of each type of exercise equipment or machine must have clear floor space of at least 30 by 48 inches and be served by an accessible route. If the clear space is enclosed on three sides (e.g., by walls or the equipment itself), the clear space must be at least 36 by 48 inches.

Most strength training equipment and machines would be considered different types. For example, a bench press machine is different from a biceps curl machine. If operators provide both a biceps curl machine and free weights, both must meet the guidelines in this section even though both can be used to strengthen biceps. Likewise, cardiovascular exercise machines, such as stationary bicycles, rowing machines, stair climbers, and treadmills, are all different types of machines. If the only difference in pieces of equipment provided is that they have different manufacturers, but are the same type, only one must comply.

Clear floor space must be positioned to allow a person to transfer from a wheelchair or to use the equipment while seated in a wheelchair. For example, to make a shoulder press accessible, the clear floor space should be next to the seat. But the clear floor space for a bench press designed for use by a person using a wheelchair would be centered on the operating mechanisms. Clear floor space for more than one piece of equipment may overlap. For example, where different types of exercise equipment and machines are located next to other pieces of equipment, the clear space may be shared. (See figure "Clear space requirements around exercise equipment" on page 171.)

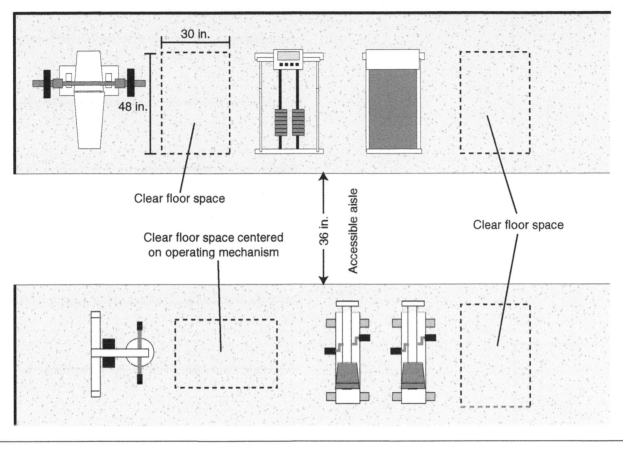

Clear space requirements around exercise equipment.

The exercise equipment and machines themselves do not need to comply with the ADAAG requirements regarding controls and operating mechanisms.

Designers and operators are encouraged to select exercise equipment that provides fitness opportunities for persons with lower body extremity disabilities.

SHOOTING FACILITIES

If facilities provide fixed firing positions, at least 5 percent, but not less than one of each type of fixed firing position, must be served by an accessible route. Fixed firing positions, must have a 60-inch diameter space with slopes not steeper than 1:48 so a wheelchair user can turn around and have a level place from which to shoot.

Types of different firing positions include positions with different admission prices, positions with or without weather covering or lighting, and positions that support different shooting events (e.g., muzzle loading rifle, small bore rifle, high power rifle, bull's eye pistol, action pistol, silhouette, trap, skeet, and archery).

BOWLING LANES

At least 5 percent, but not less than one, of each type of bowling lane must be accessible. (See page 172.) Unlike other areas of sport activity, only those team or player seating areas that serve accessible lanes must be connected with an accessible route and comply with seating requirements. Spectator seating in bowling facilities is addressed in ADAAG and will require wheelchair spaces, companion seating, and designated aisle seats.

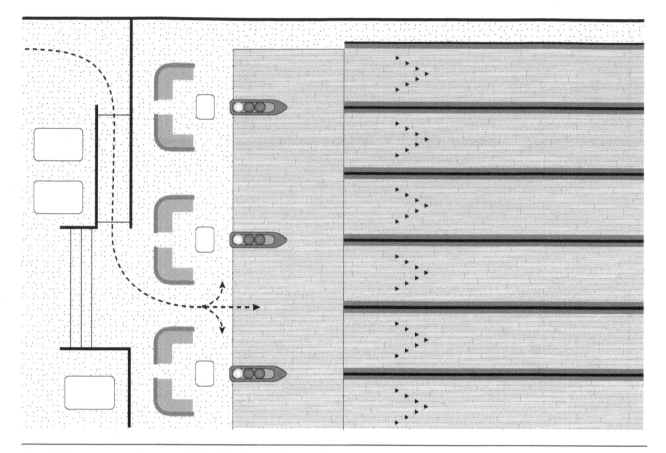

Accessible route connecting accessible bowling lanes and team player areas.

MORE INFORMATION

You can obtain copies of the recreation facility guidelines, which include sports facilities, and further technical assistance from the U.S. Access Board at www.access-board.gov, 1-800-872-2253, or 1-800-993-2822 (TTY).

Accessible Swimming Pools and Spas

A Summary of Accessibility Guidelines for Recreation Facilities

INTRODUCTION

The Americans with Disabilities Act (ADA) is a comprehensive civil rights law that prohibits discrimination on the basis of disability. The ADA requires that newly constructed and altered state and local government facilities, places of public accommodation, and commercial facilities be readily accessible to, and usable by, individuals with disabilities. The ADA Accessibility Guidelines (ADAAG) is the standard applied to buildings and facilities. Recreational facilities, including swimming pools, wading pools, and spas, are among the facilities required to comply with the ADA.

The Access Board issued accessibility guidelines for newly constructed and altered recreation facilities in 2002. The recreation facility guidelines are a supplement to ADAAG. As a supplement, they must be used in conjunction with ADAAG. References to ADAAG are mentioned throughout this summary. Copies of ADAAG and the recreation facility accessibility guidelines can be obtained through the Board's website at www.access-board.gov or by calling 1-800-872-2253 or 1-800-993-2822 (TTY).

Once these guidelines are adopted by the Department of Justice (DOJ), all newly designed, constructed, and altered recreation facilities covered by the ADA will be required to comply.

The recreation facility guidelines cover the following facilities and elements:

- Amusement rides
- Boating facilities
- Bowling lanes
- Exercise equipment
- Fishing piers and platforms
- Golf courses
- Miniature golf courses
- Shooting facilities
- Swimming pools, wading pools, and spas

This guide is intended to help designers and operators in using the accessibility guidelines for swimming pools, wading pools, and spas. These guidelines establish minimum accessibility requirements for newly designed or newly constructed and altered swimming pools, wading pools, and spas. This guide is not a collection of swimming pool or spa designs. Rather, it provides specifications for elements within a swimming pool or spa to create

Material in appendix E appears courtesy of United States Access Board.

▶ **173**

a general level of usability for individuals with disabilities. Emphasis is placed on ensuring that individuals with disabilities are generally able to access swimming pools and spas and use a variety of elements. Designers and operators are encouraged to exceed the guidelines where possible to provide increased accessibility and opportunities. Incorporating accessibility into the design of a swimming pool or spa should begin early in the planning process with careful consideration to the accessible routes and means of entry into the water.

The recreation facility guidelines were developed with significant public participation. In 1993, the Access Board established an advisory committee of 27 members to recommend accessibility guidelines for recreation facilities. The Recreation Access Advisory Committee represented the following groups and associations:

- American Ski Federation
- American Society for Testing and Materials (Public Playground Safety Committee)
- American Society of Landscape Architects
- Beneficial Designs
- City and County of San Francisco, California, Department of Public Works
- Disabled American Veterans
- Environmental Access
- Golf Course Superintendents Association of America
- Hawaii Disability and Communication Access Board
- International Association of Amusement Parks and Attractions
- Katherine McGuinness and Associates
- Lehman, Smith, and Wiseman Associates
- Michigan Department of Natural Resources
- National Council on Independent Living
- National Park Service
- National Recreation and Park Association
- New Jersey Department of Community Affairs
- Outdoor Amusement Business Association
- Paralyzed Veterans of America
- Professional Golfer Association
- Self Help for Hard of Hearing People
- States Organization for Boating Access
- Universal Studios
- U.S. Army Corps of Engineers

- U.S. Forest Service
- Y.M.C.A. of the U.S.A.
- Walt Disney Imagineering

The public was given an opportunity to comment on the recommended accessibility guidelines, and the Access Board made changes to the recommended guidelines based on the public comments. A notice of proposed rulemaking (NPRM) was published in the Federal Register in July 1999, followed by a five-month public comment period. Further input from the public was sought in July 2000 when the Access Board published a draft final rule soliciting comment. A final rule was published in September 2002.

> *"Whenever a door is closed to anyone because of a disability, we must work to open it. . . . Whenever any barrier stands between you and the full rights and dignity of citizenship, we must work to remove it, in the name of simple decency and justice. The promise of the ADA . . . has enabled people with disabilities to enjoy much greater access to a wide range of affordable travel, recreational opportunities, and life-enriching services."*
>
> —*President George W. Bush,*
> *New Freedom Initiative,*
> *February 1, 2001*

SWIMMING POOLS AND SPAS

The guidelines described in this guide focus on newly designed or newly constructed and altered swimming pools, wading pools, aquatic recreation facilities, and spas. Other provisions contained in ADAAG address elements commonly found at a swimming facility, such as accessible vehicle parking spaces, exterior accessible routes, and toilet and bathing facilities. ADAAG addresses only the built environment (structures and grounds). The guidelines do not address operational issues. Questions regarding operational issues should be directed to the Department of Justice, 1-800-514-0301 or 1-800-514-0383 (TTY).

ACCESSIBLE ROUTES

Accessible routes are continuous, unobstructed paths connecting all accessible elements and spaces of a building or facility. Accessible route requirements in ADAAG address width (minimum of 36 inches), passing space, head room, surface, slope (maximum of 1:12 or 8.33 percent), changes in level,

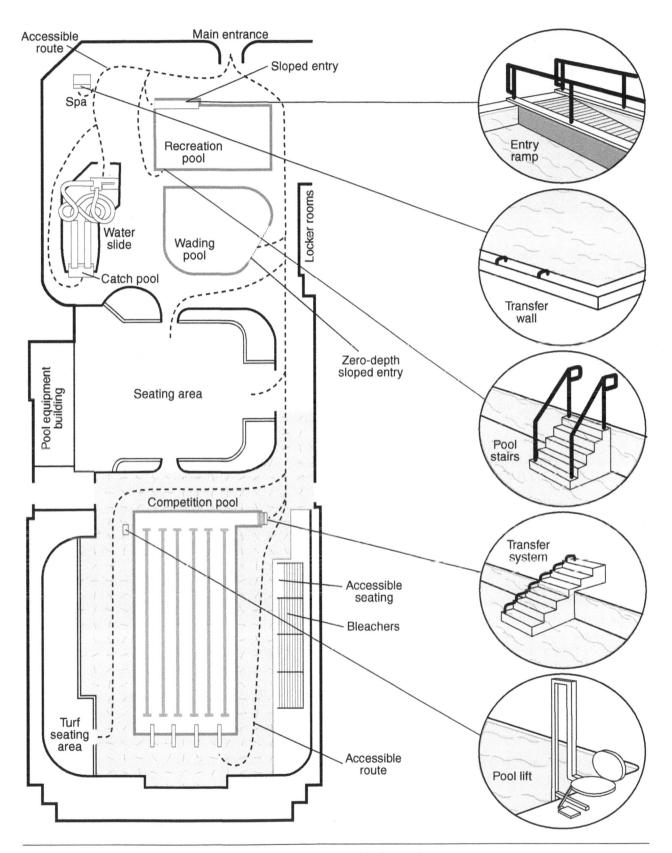

Accessible route connecting elements within a multiuse swimming pool facility.

PERMITTED MEANS OF POOL ACCESS

Pool type	Sloped entry	Lift	Transfer walls	Transfer systems	Stairs
Swimming (less than 300 linear feet of pool wall)	✓	✓			
Swimming (300 or more linear feet of pool wall)—two means of entry required	✓*	✓*	✓	✓	✓
Wave action, leisure river, and other pools where user entry is limited to one area	✓	✓		✓	
Wading pools	✓				
Spas		✓	✓	✓	

*Primary means must be by sloped entry or lift, secondary means can be any of the permitted types.

doors, egress, and areas of rescue assistance, unless modified by specific provisions outlined in this guide. An accessible route is required to provide access to the swimming areas and all the supporting amenities. An accessible route is not required to serve raised diving boards, platforms, or water slides.

TYPES OF FACILITIES AND REQUIRED MEANS OF ENTRY INTO THE WATER

Swimming Pools

Large pools must have a minimum of two accessible means of entry. A large pool is defined as any pool with over 300 linear feet of pool wall. Pool walls at diving areas and in areas where swimmers cannot enter because of landscaping or adjacent structures are still counted as part of the pool's total linear feet.

The primary means of entry must be either a sloped entry into the water or a pool lift that is capable of being independently operated by a person with a disability. The secondary means of entry could be a pool lift, sloped entry, transfer wall, transfer system, or pool stairs. It is recommended that where two means of entry are provided, they be different types and be situated on different pool walls.

Pools with less than 300 linear feet of pool wall are only required to provide one accessible means of entry, which must be either a pool lift or sloped entry.

Aquatic Recreation Facilities

Wave action pools, leisure rivers, sand bottom pools, and other pools where access to the water is limited to one area and where everyone gets in

and out at the same place, must provide at least one accessible means of entry, no matter how many linear feet of pool wall is provided. The accessible means of entry can be either a pool lift, sloped entry, or transfer system.

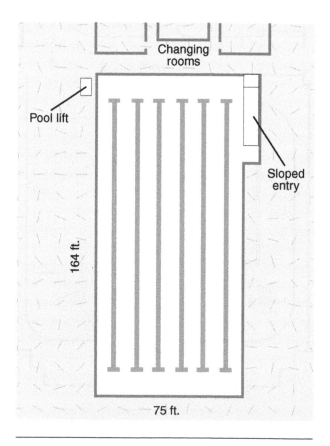

Two means of access required in larger pool.

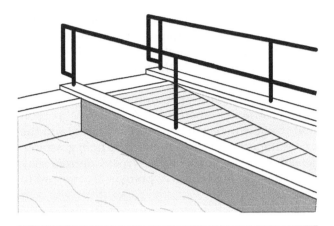

Zero-grade sloped entry into wave-action pool.

Catch Pools

A catch pool is a body of water where water slide flumes drop users into the water. An accessible means of entry or exit is not required into the catch pool. However, an accessible route must connect to the edge of the catch pool.

Wading Pools

A wading pool is a pool designed for shallow depth and is used for wading. Each wading pool must provide at least one sloped entry into the deepest part. Other forms of entry may be provided as long as a sloped entry is provided. The sloped entries for wading pools are not required to have handrails.

Spas

Spas must provide at least one accessible means of entry, which can be a pool lift, transfer wall, or transfer system. If spas are provided in a cluster, 5 percent of the total—or at least one spa—must be accessible. If there is more than one cluster, one spa or 5 percent per cluster must be accessible.

Footrests are not required on pool lifts provided at spas. However, footrests or retractable leg supports are encouraged, especially on lifts used in larger spas, where the water depth is 34 inches or more and there is sufficient space.

TYPES OF ACCESSIBLE MEANS OF ENTRY INTO THE WATER

Pool Lifts

Pool lifts must be located where the water level is not deeper than 48 inches. This provides the opportunity for someone to provide assistance from a standing position in the water if desired. If multiple pool lift locations are provided, only one must be where the water is less than 48 inches. If the entire pool is deeper than 48 inches, an exception allows operators to use a pool lift in any location as an accessible means of entry.

Seats

There are a variety of seats available on pool lifts and these guidelines do not specify the type of material or the type of seat required. However, lift seats must be a minimum of 16 inches wide. In the raised (load) position, the centerline of the seat must be located over the deck, a minimum of 16 inches from the edge of the pool. The deck surface between the centerline of the seat and the pool edge cannot have a slope greater than 1:48.

Although not required, seats with backs will enable a larger number of persons with disabilities to use the lift independently. Pool lift seats made of materials that resist corrosion, that provide a firm base, and that are padded are more usable. Headrests, seat belts, and additional leg support may also enhance accessibility and accommodate a wider variety of people with disabilities.

Clear Deck Space

Clear deck space must be provided to enable a person to get close enough to the pool lift seat to easily transfer from a wheelchair or mobility device. This clear deck space will ensure an unobstructed area for transfers between a mobility device and the seat. The clear deck space must be a minimum of 36 inches wide and extend forward a minimum of 48 inches from a line located 12 inches behind the

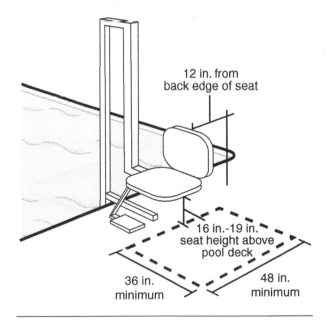

12 in. from back edge of seat

16 in.-19 in. seat height above pool deck

36 in. minimum

48 in. minimum

Pool lift.

rear edge of the seat. This space must be located on the side of the seat opposite the water. The slope of the clear deck space must not be greater than 1:48 (2 percent). This virtually flat area will make the transfer easier and safer, while still allowing water to drain away from the deck.

Seat Height

The lift must be designed so that the seat will make a stop between a minimum of 16 inches and maximum of 19 inches (measured from the deck to the top of the seat surface, when the seat is in the raised position). Lifts can provide additional stops at various heights to accommodate users of all ages and abilities.

Footrests and Armrests

Footrests and armrests provide stability for the person using the pool lift. Footrests must be provided on pool lifts, and must move together with the seat. Padding on footrests—large enough to support the whole foot—reduces the chance of injury.

Armrests are not required; however if provided, the armrest opposite the water must be removable or be able to fold clear of the seat when the seat is in the raised (load) position. This clearance is needed for people transferring between the lift and a mobility device.

Operation

Lifts must be designed and placed so that people can use them without assistance, although assistance can be provided if needed. A person must be able to call the lift when it is in either the deck or water position. It is especially important for someone who is swimming alone to be able to call the lift so she or he won't be stranded in the water for an extended period of time.

The controls and operating mechanisms must be unobstructed when a lift is in use. A person must be able to use the lift with one hand, and the operating controls must not require tight grasping, pinching, or twisting of the wrist. Controls may not require more than five pounds of pressure to operate.

Submerged Depth

Lifts must be designed so that the seat will submerge to a minimum of 18 inches below the stationary water level. This will ensure buoyancy for the person on the lift and make it easier to enter or exit.

Lifting Capacity

Lifts must have the capability of supporting a minimum weight of 300 pounds and be capable of sustaining a static load that is at least 1.5 times the rated load. Where possible, lifts that can support a greater weight capacity are encouraged.

SLOPED ENTRIES

Sloped entries must comply with ADAAG accessible route provisions (36 inch minimum width, maximum 1:12 or 8.33 percent slope), except that the surface does not need to be slip resistant. The slope may be designed as zero grade beach or ramp access. With either design, the maximum slope permitted is 1:12 (8.33 percent).

In most cases, it is not appropriate to submerge personal wheelchairs and mobility devices in water. Some have batteries, motors, and electrical systems that can be damaged or contaminate the pool. Facilities that use sloped entries are encouraged to provide an aquatic wheelchair designed for access into the water. Persons transfer to the aquatic wheelchair and access the water using it, leaving their personal mobility device on the deck. Operators and facility managers may need to consider storage options for personal mobility devices if deck space is limited.

Submerged Depth

Sloped entries must extend to a depth between 24 inches minimum and 30 inches maximum below the stationary water level. This depth is necessary for individuals using the sloped entry to become buoyant. Where the sloped entry has a running slope greater than 1:20 (5 percent), a landing at both the

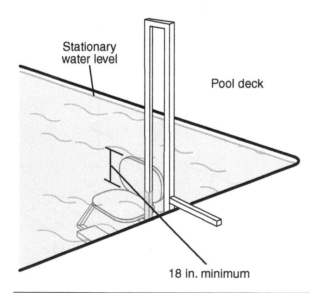

Pool lift submerged depth.

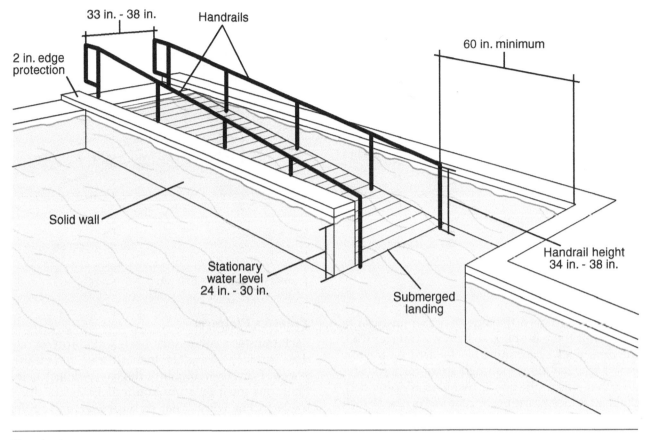

Sloped entry ramp.

top and bottom of the ramp is required. At least one landing must be located between 24 and 30 inches below the stationary water level. Landings must be a minimum of 36 inches in width and 60 inches in length. The sloped entry may be a maximum of 30 feet at 1:12 (8.33%) slope before an intermediate landing is required. Adding a solid wall on the side closest to the water can enhance safety.

Handrails

Sloped entries must have handrails on both sides regardless of the slope. Handrail extensions are required at the top landing but not at the bottom. The clear width between handrails must be between 33 and 38 inches. The handrail height must be between 34 and 48 inches to the top of the gripping surface. This provision does not require the handrails to be below the stationary water level, which could be considered an underwater obstruction. No minimum width is required between handrails provided on sloped entries that serve wave action pools, leisure rivers, sand bottom pools, and other pools where people can enter only in one place. Handrails are required to comply with ADAAG provisions (diameter, non-rotating, and height).

TRANSFER WALLS

A transfer wall is a wall along an accessible route that allows a person to leave a mobility device and transfer onto the wall and then into a pool or spa.

Grab Bars

Transfer walls must have at least one grab bar. Grab bars must be perpendicular to the pool wall and extend the full width of the wall so a person can use them for support into the water. The top of the gripping surface must be 4 to 6 inches above the wall to provide leverage to the person using the bars. If only one bar is provided, the clearance must be a minimum of 24 inches on each side of the bar. If two bars are provided, the clearance must be a minimum of 24 inches between the bars. The diameter of the grab bars must comply with ADAAG (diameter between 1.25 and 1.5 inches, not abrasive, and non-rotating).

Clear Deck Space

Clear deck space of 60 by 60 inches minimum, with a slope of not more than 1:48, must be provided at the base of a transfer wall. This will allow persons using a wheelchair to turn around and access the

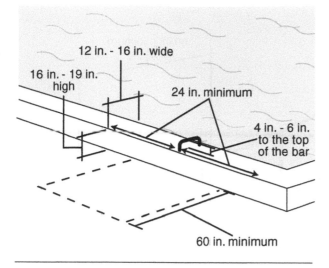

Transfer wall with one grab bar.

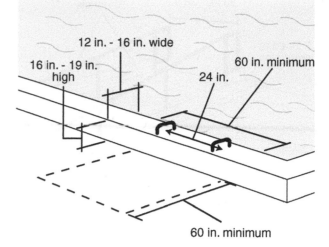

Transfer wall with two grab bars.

wall, depending on the side they can best use to transfer. If there is one grab bar on a transfer wall, the clear deck space must be centered on the one grab bar. That allows enough space for a transfer on either side of the bar. If two bars are provided, the clear deck space must be centered on the 24-inch clearance between the two bars.

Height

The transfer wall height must be 16 inches minimum to 19 inches maximum, measured from the deck.

Width and Length

Transfer walls must be a minimum of 12 inches wide to a maximum of 16 inches wide. This provides enough space for a person to sit comfortably on the surface of the wall and pivot to access the water. The wall must be a minimum of 60 inches long and must be centered on the clear deck space. Additional length will provide increased space and options for transferring.

Surface

Since people using transfer walls are in bathing suits, their skin may be in contact with the wall. To prevent injuries, the wall surface must have rounded edges and not be sharp.

TRANSFER SYSTEMS

A transfer system consists of a transfer platform and a series of transfer steps that descend into the water. Users need to transfer from their wheelchair or mobility device to the transfer platform and continue transferring into the water, step by step, bumping their way in or out of the pool.

Transfer Platform

Each transfer system must have a platform on the deck surface so users can maneuver on and off the system from their mobility device or wheelchair. Platforms must be a minimum of 19 inches deep by 24 inches wide. That provides enough room for a person transferring to maintain balance and provides enough space to maneuver on top of it.

Platform Height

Transfer platforms must be between 16 and 19 inches high, measured from the deck.

Clear Deck Space

The base of the transfer platform must have a clear deck space adjacent to it that is 60 by 60 inches minimum, with a slope not steeper than 1:48 so a person using a wheelchair can turn around and maneuver into transfer position. The space must be centered along the 24-inch minimum unobstructed side of the transfer platform. A level, unobstructed space will help a person transferring from a mobility device.

Transfer Steps

The maximum height of transfer steps is 8 inches, although shorter heights are recommended. Each transfer step must have a tread depth of 14 inches minimum to 17 inches maximum and a minimum tread width of 24 inches. The steps must extend into the water a minimum of 18 inches below the stationary water level.

Surface

The surface of the transfer platform and steps must not be sharp and must have rounded edges to prevent injuries.

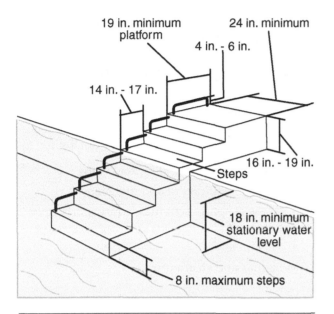

Transfer system platform and steps.

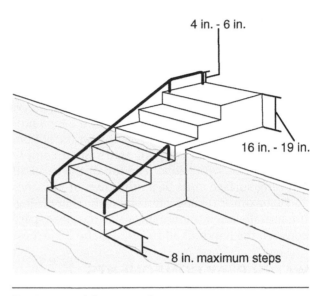

Continuous grab bar at transfer system.

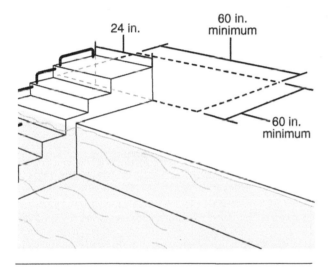

Clear deck space located at a transfer system.

Grab Bars

A grab bar must be provided on at least one side of each step and on the transfer platform, or as a continuous grab bar serving each step and the platform. The bar must not obstruct transfer onto the platform. If a grab bar is provided on each step, the top of the gripping surface must be 4 inches minimum to 6 inches maximum above each step. If a continuous bar is provided, the top of the gripping surface must be 4 inches minimum to 6 inches maximum above each step nosing. Grab bars on transfer systems must comply with ADAAG (diameter between 1.25 and 1.5 inches, not abrasive, and non-rotating).

ACCESSIBLE POOL STAIRS

Accessible pool stairs are designed to provide assistance with balance and support from a standing position when moving from the pool deck into the water and out. ADAAG provisions for stairs include the requirement that all steps have uniform riser heights and uniform tread widths of not less than 11 inches, measured from riser to riser. Additionally, open risers are not permitted. Other stairs or steps provided in the pool are not required to meet these guidelines.

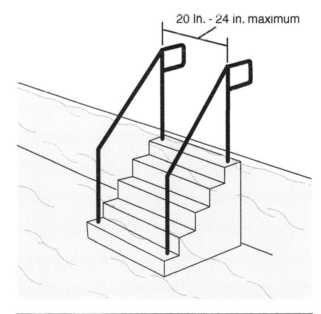

Pool stairs.

Handrails

Pool stairs must have handrails with a minimum width between the rails of 20 inches and a maximum of 24 inches. The 20- to 24-inch width for the accessible pool stairs is intended to provide support for individuals with disabilities who are ambulatory. Handrail extensions are required on the top landing of the stairs but are not required at the bottom landing. Handrails on pool stairs must comply with ADAAG provisions. The top of the handrail gripping surface must be a minimum of 34 inches and a maximum of 38 inches above the stair nosing. If handrails are mounted on walls, the clear space between the handrail and wall must be 1.5 inches.

WATER PLAY COMPONENTS

If water play components are provided, they must comply with the Access Board's Play Area Guidelines and accessible route provisions.

If the surface of the accessible route, clear floor or ground spaces, and turning spaces that connect play components are submerged, the accessible route does not have to comply with the requirements for cross slope, running slope, and surface conditions.

Transfer systems may be used instead of ramps to connect elevated water play components.

OTHER ACCESSIBLE ELEMENTS

If swimming pools are part of a multiuse facility, designers and operators must also comply with ADAAG and all applicable requirements for recreation facilities. These include, but are not limited to:

- Dressing, fitting, and locker rooms
- Exercise equipment and machines
- Areas of sports activities (court sports, sports fields, etc.)
- Play areas
- Saunas and steam rooms

MORE INFORMATION

You can obtain copies of the recreation facility guidelines, which include swimming pools, wading pools, and spas, and further technical assistance from the U.S. Access Board at www.access-board.gov, 1-800-872-2253, or 1-800-993-2822 (TTY).

Trade and Professional Associations Involved in the Health/Fitness Facility Industry

Aerobics and Fitness Association of America
15250 Ventura Boulevard, Suite 200
Sherman Oaks, CA 91403
877-968-7263
www.afaa.com

**American Alliance for Health, Physical
 Education, Recreation and Dance**
1900 Association Drive
Reston, VA 20191-1598
800-213-7193
www.aahperd.org

**American Association of Cardiovascular
 and Pulmonary Rehabilitation**
401 N. Michigan Avenue, Suite 2200
Chicago, IL 60611
312-321-5146
www.aacvpr.org

American College of Sports Medicine
401 W. Michigan Street
P.O. Box 1440
Indianapolis, IN 46206-1440
317-637-9200
www.acsm.org

American Council on Exercise
4851 Paramount Drive
San Diego, CA 92123
888-825-3636
www.acefitness.org

American Heart Association
7272 Greenville Avenue
Dallas, TX 75231
800-242-8721
www.americanheart.org

American Massage Therapy Association
500 Davis Street, Suite 900
Evanston, IL 60201-4695
877-905-0577
www.amtamassage.org

IDEA Health and Fitness Association
10455 Pacific Center Court
San Diego, CA 92121-4339
800-999-4332, ext. 7
www.ideafit.com

International Council on Active Aging
3307 Trutch Street
Vancouver, BC V6L-2T3
Canada
866-335-9777
www.icaa.cc

International Health, Racquet and Sportsclub
    Association
70 Fargo Street
Boston, MA 02210
800-228-4772
www.ihrsa.org

Medical Fitness Association
1905 Huguenot Road, Suite 203
P.O. Box 73103
Richmond, VA 23235-8026
804-897-5701
www.medicalfitness.org

National Athletic Trainers' Association
2952 Stemmons Freeway #200
Dallas, TX 75247
214-637-6282
www.nata.org

National Center on Physical Activity and
    Disability
1640 W. Roosevelt Road
Chicago, IL 60608-6904
800-900-8086
www.ncpad.org

National Institute for Occupational Safety
    and Health
Patriots Plaza Building
395 E. Street, SW, Suite 9200
Washington, DC 20201
800-232-4636
www.cdc.gov/niosh

National Strength and Conditioning Association
1885 Bob Johnson Drive
Colorado Springs, CO 80906
800-815-6826
www.nsca-lift.org

National Swimming Pool Foundation
4775 Granby Circle
Colorado Springs, CO 80919
719-540-9119
www.nspf.com

National Wellness Institute
1300 College Court
P.O. Box 827
Stevens Point, WI 54481
800-243-8694
www.nationalwellness.org

President's Council on Fitness, Sports and
    Nutrition
1101 Wootton Parkway, Suite 560
Rockville, MD 20852
240-276-9567
www.fitness.gov

Sporting Goods Manufacturers Association
8505 Fenton Street, Suite 211
Silver Spring, MD 20910
301-495-6321
www.sgma.com

U.S. Squash Racquets Association
555 Eighth Avenue, Suite 1102
New York, NY 10018-4311
212-268-4090
www.us-squash.org

The Wellness Council of America
17002 Marcy Street, Suite 140
Omaha, NE 68118
402-827-3590
www.welcoa.org

About the American College of Sports Medicine

"Advancing health through science, education and medicine."

This simple statement describes a complex organization working to improve quality of life in more than 80 countries. The American College of Sports Medicine is more than 20,000 professionals practicing clinical medicine, research, education, and an array of health and fitness disciplines.

The world's largest organization of its kind, ACSM tackles issues as diverse as obesity and motorsport injuries. The College is at the nexus of science and public policy, working to develop new knowledge and apply it toward a healthier, more fit society. From astronauts to student-athletes, physiologists to personal trainers, people turn to ACSM for definitive information on health, fitness, sports medicine, and exercise science. Founded in 1954, ACSM is internationally regarded as defining the gold standard for science, education, and certification.

ACSM reaches professionals and the public through a variety of means:

- Periodicals such as *Medicine & Science in Sports & Exercise*®*, Sports Medicine Bulletin, Exercise and Sport Sciences Reviews, ACSM's Health & Fitness Journal*®, *Current Sports Medicine Reports,* and the online consumer newsletter *ACSM Fit Society*® Page.

- The ACSM website, www.acsm.org, serves as a portal to health and fitness information, science-based guidance, professional development, and other resources.

- Meetings present the latest scientific research and practical and clinical applications as well as fitness techniques and public health issues.

- Through media outreach, ACSM experts provide accurate, evidence-based insight into sports medicine, exercise science, and health and fitness.

- Books, pamphlets, and other publications present consumer advice, standards, and guidelines for practitioners, and other definitive information.

- ACSM has a presence on Facebook, Twitter, and YouTube.

ACSM MEMBERSHIP

The American College of Sports Medicine is a lifelong resource, serving student members and working professionals in more than 50 occupations. ACSM membership brings a host of benefits, such as publications, conferences, and regional chapter services. Members enjoy special discounts and opportunities.

Membership categories include the following:

- Professional member (degreed or working in a relevant field)
- Professional-in-training member (in residency or postdoctoral fellowship)
- Graduate student member
- Undergraduate student member

- ACSM's Alliance of Health and Fitness Professionals (professionals or students in the health and fitness and medical fitness industries)

And, in recognition of their distinguished achievement and service to the profession, members can pursue the status of Fellow in the American College of Sports Medicine.

As professionals in training, students are an important focus of ACSM. The board of trustees includes student representation, and each Regional Chapter selects a representative to the Student Affairs Committee. Student members enjoy discounted dues, publications, and meetings. More information is available at www.acsm.org/students.

ACSM CERTIFICATION: THE GOLD STANDARD

ACSM's emphasis on rigorous science and professionalism has earned it a reputation as the gold standard for certification of health and fitness professionals. To consumers, institutions, and organizations that insist on demonstrated knowledge and skills, ACSM certification signifies the highest level of preparation and practice.

For more on ACSM certification programs, see the section "ACSM Certification Programs."

ACSM INTEREST GROUPS

Interest Groups provide a forum for focused discussion, activity, and debate among members with similar interests. Many find the networking opportunities especially valuable. Through participation in ACSM Interest Groups, members take part in the academic and professional life of the College and help advance its mission.

ACSM REGIONAL CHAPTERS

Twelve Regional Chapters allow greater participation among members and encourage networking and professional growth for longtime members and students alike. Regional Chapters produce publications and hold annual scientific meetings.

CONTACTING ACSM

www.acsm.org
401 W. Michigan Street
P.O. Box 1440
Indianapolis, IN 46206-1440
317-637-9200 (phone)
317-634-7817 (fax)

AMERICAN COLLEGE OF SPORTS MEDICINE CERTIFICATIONS FOR HEALTH AND FITNESS PROFESSIONALS

For 35 years, professionals who wish to demonstrate the highest level of expertise in exercise testing and prescription have sought ACSM certification. This gold standard distinguishes those who work in many settings:

- Hospital clinical and rehabilitation programs
- Corporate wellness centers
- Park and recreation departments
- Health and fitness facilities
- Senior residences and care programs

ACSM CERTIFICATION PROGRAMS

The American College of Sports Medicine offers the following credentials:

- ACSM Certified Group Exercise Instructor (GEI)
- ACSM Certified Personal Trainer℠ (CPT)
- ACSM Health Fitness Specialist (HFS)
- ACSM Certified Clinical Exercise Specialist (CES)
- ACSM Registered Clinical Exercise Physiologist® (RCEP)
- ACSM/NCPAD Certified Inclusive Fitness Trainer (CIFT)
- ACSM/ACS Certified Cancer Exercise Trainer (CET)
- ACSM/NSPAPPH Physical Activity in Public Health Specialist (PAPHS)

The ACSM Certified Personal Trainer℠ is a fitness professional involved in developing and implementing an individualized approach to exercise leadership in healthy populations and in those with medical clearance to exercise. Using a variety of teaching techniques, the CPT is proficient in leading and demonstrating safe and effective methods of exercise by applying the principles of exercise science. The ACSM CPT is familiar with forms of exercise used to improve, maintain, and optimize health-related components of physical fitness and performance. CPTs are proficient in writing appropriate exercise recommendations, leading and demonstrating safe and effective methods of exercise, and motivating people to begin and to continue with their healthy behaviors.

The ACSM Health Fitness Specialist is a professional qualified to assess, design, and implement individual and group exercise and fitness programs for low-risk individuals and individuals with controlled disease. The HFS is skilled in evaluating health behaviors and risk factors, conducting fitness assessments, writing appropriate exercise prescriptions, and motivating individuals to modify negative health habits and maintain positive lifestyle behaviors for health promotion.

The ACSM Registered Clinical Exercise Physiologist® (RCEP) is an allied health professional who works with persons with chronic diseases and conditions in which exercise has been shown to be beneficial. The RCEP performs health, physical activity, and fitness assessments and prescribes exercise and physical activity primarily in hospitals or other health-provider settings.

For information about each certification, visit the website at www.acsm.org/certification. Certification at a given level requires the candidate to have a knowledge and skills base commensurate with that specific level of certification. Each level of certification has minimum requirements for experience, level of education, and other certifications. "ACSM's Get Certified Guide" outlines the requirements and is available for free on the "Get Certified" page of the website.

35 YEARS OF CERTIFICATION

The ACSM certification program began in 1975 along with publication of the first edition of *ACSM's Guidelines for Exercise Testing and Prescription*. That era was marked by rapid development of exercise programs for patients with stable coronary artery disease. ACSM sought a means to disseminate accurate information on this health-care initiative through expression of consensus from its members in basic science, clinical practice, and education. These early clinical certifications helped establish safe and scientifically based exercise services for cardiac rehabilitation.

Over the past 35 years, exercise has gained widespread recognition as an important component in programs of rehabilitative care or health maintenance for an expanding list of chronic diseases and disabling conditions. The growth of public interest in the role of exercise in health promotion has been equally impressive. In addition, federal policy makers have revisited questions of medical efficacy and financing for exercise services in rehabilitative

care of selected patients. In recent years, recommendations from the U.S. Public Health Service and the U.S. Surgeon General have acknowledged the central role that regular physical activity can play in preventing disease and promoting health.

ACSM's development of the health and fitness certifications in the 1980s increased the availability of qualified professionals providing scientifically sound advice and supervision regarding physical activities in apparently healthy adults. Since 1975, ACSM has certified more than 30,000 professionals. Many colleges and universities have adopted ACSM guidelines in establishing standardized curricula that are focused on the knowledge and skills required for various certifications.

The ACSM University Connection Endorsement Program is designed to recognize institutions with educational programs that meet all of the knowledge and skills specified by the ACSM Committee on Certification and Registry Boards (CCRB).

ACSM's Certified News brings best practices and other information to certified professionals. ACSM also oversees continuing education requirements for maintenance of certification. Continuing education credits can be accrued through ACSM-sponsored educational programs such as workshops, Regional Chapter meetings and annual meetings, and other educational programs approved by the ACSM Professional Education Committee. These enhancements support the continued professional growth of those who have made a commitment to service in the health and fitness field.

HOW TO OBTAIN INFORMATION AND APPLICATION MATERIALS

ACSM certification programs are subject to continual review and revision. Content development is entrusted to a diverse committee of professional volunteers with expertise in exercise science, medicine, and program management. The committee's expertise also includes design and procedures for competency assessment. The ACSM National Center oversees administration of certification. Inquiries concerning certifications, application requirements, fees, and examination test sites and dates may be made to:

ACSM Certification Resource Center
800-486-5643
Website: www.acsm.org/certification
E-mail: certification@acsm.org

AHA/ACSM Joint Position Statement

Recommendations for Cardiovascular Screening, Staffing, and Emergency Policies at Health/Fitness Facilities

SUMMARY

The promotion of physical activity is at the top of our national public health agenda. Although regular exercise reduces subsequent cardiovascular morbidity and mortality, the incidence of a cardiovascular event during exercise in patients with cardiac disease is estimated to be 10 times that of otherwise healthy persons. Adequate screening and evaluation are important to identify and counsel persons with underlying cardiovascular disease before they begin exercising at moderate to vigorous levels. This statement provides recommendations for *cardiovascular screening* of all persons (children, adolescents, and adults) before enrollment or participation in activities at health/fitness facilities. Staff qualifications and emergency policies related to cardiovascular safety are also discussed.

INTRODUCTION

The message from the nation's scientists is clear, unequivocal, and unified: physical inactivity is a risk factor for cardiovascular disease (7,18), and its prevalence is an important public health issue. New scientific knowledge based on epidemiological observational studies, cohort studies, controlled trials, and basic research has led to an unprecedented focus on physical activity and exercise. The promotion of physical activity is at the top of our national public health agenda, as seen in the publication of the 1996 report of the U.S. Surgeon General on physical activity and health (20).

The attention now being given to physical activity supports the goals of Healthy People 2000 (10) and should lead to increased levels of regular physical activity throughout the U.S. population, including the nearly one fourth of adult Americans who have some form of cardiovascular disease (3). Although regular exercise reduces subsequent cardiovascular morbidity and mortality (7,17,18), the incidence of a cardiovascular event during exercise in patients with cardiac disease is estimated to be 10 times that of otherwise healthy persons (8). Adequate screening and evaluation are important to identify and counsel persons with underlying cardiovascular disease before they begin exercising at moderate to vigorous levels.

Moderate (or higher) levels of physical activity and exercise are achieved in a number of settings, including more than 15,000 health/fitness facilities across the country. A recent survey of 110 health/fitness facilities in Massachusetts found that efforts to screen new members at enrollment were limited and inconsistent (14). Nearly 40% of responding facilities stated that they do not routinely use a screening interview or questionnaire to evaluate new members for symptoms or history of cardiovascular disease, and 10% stated that they conducted no initial cardiovascular health history screening at all.

This statement provides recommendations for *cardiovascular screening* of all persons (children, adolescents, and adults) before enrollment or participation in activities at health/fitness facilities. Staff qualifications and emergency policies related to cardiovascular safety are also discussed. Health/fitness facilities are defined here as organizations that offer health and fitness programs as their primary or secondary service or that promote high-intensity recreational physical activity (e.g., basketball, tennis, racquetball, and swim clubs). Ideally such facilities have a professional staff, but those that provide space and equipment only (e.g., unsupervised hotel exercise rooms) are also included. A health/fitness facility user is defined as a dues-paying member or a guest paying a regular daily fee to use the facility specifically to exercise. These recommendations are intended to assist health/fitness facility staff, healthcare providers, and consumers in the promotion and performance of safe and effective physical activity/exercise.

The writing group based these recommendations on a review of the literature and the consensus of the group. Earlier statements from the American Heart Association (AHA) and the American College of Sports Medicine (ACSM) are highlighted and supplemented. These recommendations were peer reviewed by selected authorities in the field representing the AHA, the ACSM, the American College of Cardiology, the International Health Racquet and Sports Clubs Association (IHRSA), and the Young Men's Christian Association. The recommendations are not mandatory or all-encompassing, nor do they limit provision of individualized care by practitioners exercising independent judgment. With this statement the AHA and the ACSM assume no responsibility toward any individual for whom this statement may be applied in the provision of individualized care. Specific details about exercise testing and training of persons with and without cardiovascular disease and those with other health problems are provided elsewhere (2,6,8,21). The ACSM has published comprehensive guidelines for operating health/fitness facilities (19). Although issues in competitive sports are beyond the scope of this statement, the 26th Bethesda Conference (28) on sudden cardiac death in competitive athletes and the AHA (12) provide specific recommendations for the screening and evaluation of athletes for congenital heart disease, systemic hypertension, and other cardiovascular diseases before participation in competitive sports.

CARDIOVASCULAR SCREENING

Rationale

Regular exercise results in increased exercise capacity and physical fitness, which can lead to many health benefits. Persons who are physically active appear to have lower rates of all-cause mortality, probably because of a decrease in occurrence of chronic illnesses, including coronary heart disease. This benefit may be the result of an improvement in cardiovascular risk factors in addition to enhanced fibrinolysis, improved endothelial function, decreased sympathetic tone, and other as yet undetermined factors (7). Regular endurance exercise leads to favorable alterations in the cardiovascular, musculoskeletal, and neurohumoral systems. The result is a training effect, which allows an individual to do increasing amounts of work while lowering the heart rate and blood pressure response to submaximal exercise. Such an effect is particularly desirable in patients with coronary artery disease because it allows increased activity with less ischemia (7).

The Centers for Disease Control and Prevention (18), the ACSM (18), and the AHA (6) recommend that every American participate in at least moderate-intensity physical activity for ≥30 min on most, if not all, days of the week. Unfortunately, many Americans are sedentary or perform too little physical activity; only 22% of adult Americans engage in regular exercise ≥5 times a week (20). The prevalence of physical inactivity is higher among culturally diverse segments of the U.S. population, low-income groups, the elderly, and women (20). It is important for healthcare providers to educate the public about the benefits of physical activity and to encourage more leisure-time exercise, particularly for those who are underactive. Consumers should seek information about safe and effective ways to increase physical activity and initiate and maintain a regular program of exercise.

Efforts to promote physical activity will result in an increasing number of persons with and without heart disease joining the more than 20 million persons who already exercise at health/fitness facilities (16). Current market research indicates that 50% of health/fitness facility members are older than 35 yr, and the fastest-growing segments of users are those older than 55 yr and those aged 35-54 yr (16). With increased physical activity, more people with symptoms of or known cardiovascular disease will face the cardiovascular stress of physical activity and possible risk of a cardiac event. More than one fourth of all Americans have some form of cardiovascular disease (3). The prevalence of coronary heart disease for American adults aged 20 yr and older is 7.2% in the general population, 7.5% for non-Hispanic whites, 6.9% for non-Hispanic blacks, and 5.6% for Mexican Americans (3). The prevalence of myocardial infarction in older Americans aged 65-69 yr is 18.0% for men and 9.7% for women (3).

Moderately strenuous physical exertion may trigger ischemic cardiac events, particularly among persons not accustomed to regular physical activity and exercise. Siscovick et al. (23) examined the incidence of primary cardiac arrest in men aged 25-75 yr after excluding those with a history of clinically recognized heart disease. Although the risk was significantly increased during high-intensity exercise, the likelihood for primary cardiac arrest during such activity in a clinically healthy population was estimated at 0.55 events/10,000 men per year. Maron et al. (13) studied causes of sudden death in competitive athletes. In persons younger than 35 yr, 48% of deaths were due to hypertrophic cardiomyopathy. Coronary artery anomalies, idiopathic left ventricular hypertrophy, and coronary heart disease each accounted for 10-20% of deaths. In those over 35, coronary artery disease accounted for approximately 80% of all deaths. Overall, the absolute incidence of death during exercise in the general population is low (25,26,29). *Each year approximately 0.75 and 0.13/100,000 young male and female athletes (29) and 6/100,000 middle-aged men die during exertion (25).* No estimates are available for middle-aged women or the elderly.

Cardiovascular events other than death during exercise have also been studied. Data from the Framingham heart study indicate that the baseline risk of myocardial infarction in a 50-yr-old man who is a nonsmoker and does not have diabetes is approximately 1% per year, or approximately 1 chance per million per hour (4). Heavy exertion [≥6 METs (metabolic equivalents)] within 1 h of symptomatic onset of acute myocardial infarction has been reported in 4.4-7.1% of patients (15,31). The adjusted relative risk is significantly greater in persons who do not participate in regular physical activity, with an approximate threefold increase in risk during the morning hours. The relation of physical activity to acute myocardial infarction in the thrombolytic era was examined among 3,339 patients in the TIMI II trial (27), in which moderate or marked physical activity preceded myocardial infarction in 18.7% of patients.

Van Camp et al. (30) reported the incidence of major cardiovascular complications in 167 randomly selected cardiac rehabilitation programs that provided supervised exercise training to 51,000 patients with known cardiovascular disease. The incidence of myocardial infarction was 1 per 294,000 person-hours; the incidence of death was 1 per 784,000 person-hours.

Screening Prospective Members/Users

All facilities offering exercise equipment or services should conduct cardiovascular screening of all new members and/or prospective users. The primary purpose of preparticipation screening is to identify both those not known to be at risk and those known to be at risk for a cardiovascular event during exercise. Recent evidence suggests that screening by health/fitness facilities is done only sporadically (14). In Canada, evidence from the Canadian Home Fitness test and its screening instrument, the Physical Activity Readiness Questionnaire (PAR-Q), suggests that even simple screening questionnaires can effectively identify many persons at high risk and increase the safety of nonsupervised exercise (22). Current knowledge of the relation between identifiable risk factors, the incidence of cardiovascular disease, and the triggering factors for acute myocardial infarction suggests that screening is both reasonable and prudent.

The cost-effectiveness of preparticipation screening is an important consideration. Exercise testing is comparatively expensive. The incidence of false-positive findings when testing asymptomatic persons (9) and the need to follow up abnormal results can lead to subsequent and more costly procedures. A thorough and mandatory screening process that might prove optimally sensitive in detecting occult cardiovascular disease might be so prohibitive to participation that fewer persons would engage in a fitness program. Such a result would be counterproductive to the goal of maximizing physical activity. Because most of the health benefits of exercise accrue at moderate levels of intensity (18), in which the risks are probably low, recommendations that would inhibit large numbers of persons from participating in exercise programs are not justified. Preparticipation screening should identify persons at high risk and should be simple and easy to perform. Public health efforts should focus on increasing the use of preparticipation screening.

Two practical tools for preparticipation screening are likely to have an effect on identifying high-risk individuals without inhibiting their participation in exercise programs. The PAR-Q (24) (Table 1) is a self-administered questionnaire that focuses primarily on symptoms that might suggest angina pectoris. Participants are directed to contact their personal physician if they answer "yes" to ≥1 questions. The PAR-Q also identifies musculoskeletal problems that should be evaluated before participation because these might involve modification of the exercise program. The questionnaire is designed to be completed when the participant registers at

TABLE 1	Revised Physical Activity Readiness Questionnaire (PAR-Q)

Yes   No

___ ___ **1.** Has a doctor ever said that you have a heart condition and recommended only medically supervised activity?

___ ___ **2.** Do you have chest pain brought on by physical activity?

___ ___ **3.** Have you developed chest pain in the past month?

___ ___ **4.** Have you on one or more occasions lost consciousness or fallen over as a result of dizziness?

___ ___ **5.** Do you have a bone or joint problem that could be aggravated by the proposed physical activity?

___ ___ **6.** Has a doctor ever recommended medication for your blood pressure or a heart condition?

___ ___ **7.** Are you aware, through your own experience or a doctor's advice, of any other physical reason that would prohibit you from exercising without medical supervision?

If you answer "yes" to any of these questions, call your personal physician or healthcare provider before increasing your physical activity.

Adapted from Shephard et al. (22) and Thomas et al. (24).

a health/fitness facility. In unsupervised fitness facilities (e.g., hotel fitness centers), the PAR-Q can be self-administered by means of signs prominently displayed at the main entry into the facility. Although less satisfactory than documenting the results of screening, use of signs and similar visual methods are a minimal recommendation for encouraging prospective users to assess their health risks while exercising at any facility.

Another simple, self-administered device that aims to identify high-risk individuals without negatively impacting participation is a questionnaire patterned after one developed by the Wisconsin Affiliate of the American Heart Association (11) (Table 2). The one-page form is slightly more complex than the PAR-Q and uses history, symptoms, and risk factors (including age) to direct prospective members to either participate in an exercise program or contact their physician (or appropriate healthcare provider) before participation. Persons at higher risk are directed to seek facilities providing appropriate levels of staff supervision. The questionnaire can be administered within a few minutes on the same form participants use to join or register at the facility. It identifies potentially high-risk participants, documents the results of screening, educates the consumer, and encourages and fosters appropriate use of the healthcare system. In addition, it can guide staff qualifications and requirements. This instrument is also simple enough to be adapted for use as self-screening signs posted in nonstaffed facilities.

Health appraisal questionnaires should preferably be interpreted by qualified staff (see next section for criteria) who can limit the number of unnecessary referrals for preparticipation medical evaluation, avoiding undue expense and barriers to participation.

In view of the potential legal risk assumed by operators of health/fitness facilities, it is recommended that all facilities providing staff supervision document the results of screening. Screening, particularly for participants for whom a medical evaluation is recommended, requires time, personnel, and financial resources. Individual facilities can determine the most cost-effective way to conduct and document preparticipation screening.

Every effort should be made to educate all prospective new members about the importance of obtaining a health appraisal and—*if indicated*—medical evaluation/recommendation before beginning exercise testing/training. The potential risks inherent in not obtaining an appraisal should also be emphasized. Without an appraisal, it is impossible

TABLE 2 AHA/ACSM Health/Fitness Facility Preparticipation Screening Questionnaire

Assess your health needs by marking all *true* statements.

History

You have had:

_____ heart attack

_____ heart surgery

_____ cardiac catheterization

_____ pacemaker/implantable cardiac defibrillator/rhythm disturbance

_____ heart valve disease

_____ heart failure

_____ heart transplantation

_____ congenital heart disease

If you marked any of the statements in this section, consult your healthcare provider before engaging in exercise. You may need to use a facility with a medically **qualified staff.**

Symptoms

_____ You experience chest discomfort with exertion.

_____ You experience unreasonable breathlessness.

_____ You experience dizziness, fainting, blackouts.

_____ You take heart medications.

Other health issues

_____ You have musculoskeletal problems.

_____ You have concerns about the safety of exercise.

_____ You take prescription medication(s).

_____ You are pregnant.

Cardiovascular risk factors

_____ You are a man older than 45 years.

_____ You are a woman older than 55 years or you have had a hysterectomy or you are postmenopausal.

_____ You smoke.

_____ Your blood pressure is greater than 140/90.

_____ You don't know your blood pressure.

_____ You take blood pressure medication.

_____ Your blood cholesterol level is >240 mg/dL.

If you marked two or more of the statements in this section, you should consult your healthcare provider before engaging in exercise. You might benefit by using a facility with a **professionally qualified exercise staff** *to guide your exercise program.*

_____ You don't know your cholesterol level.

_____ You have a close blood relative who had a heart attack before age 55 (father or brother) or age 65 (mother or sister).

_____ You are diabetic or take medicine to control your blood sugar.

_____ You are physically inactive (i.e., you get less than 30 minutes of physical activity on at least 3 days per week).

_____ You are more than 20 pounds overweight.

_____ None of the above is true.

You should be able to exercise safely without consulting your healthcare provider in almost any facility that meets your exercise program needs.

AHA/ACSM indicates American Heart Association/American College of Sports Medicine.

to determine whether a person may be at significant risk of severe bodily harm or death by participating in an exercise program. The same is true of persons who undergo a health appraisal, are identified as having symptoms of or known cardiovascular disease, and refuse or neglect to obtain the recommended medical evaluation yet seek admission to a health/fitness facility program. *Due to safety concerns, persons with known cardiovascular disease who do not obtain recommended medical evaluations and those who fail to complete the health appraisal questionnaire upon request may be excluded from participation in a health/fitness facility exercise program to the extent permitted by law.*

Persons without symptoms or a known history of cardiovascular disease who do not obtain the recommended medical evaluation after completing a health appraisal should be required to sign an assumption of risk or release/waiver. Both of these forms may be legally recognized in the jurisdiction where the facility is located. When appropriate guidelines are followed, it is likely that the potential benefits of physical activity will outweigh the risks. *Persons without symptoms or a known history of cardiovascular disease who do not obtain recommended medical evaluations or sign a release/waiver upon request may be excluded from participation in a health/fitness facility exercise program to the extent permitted by law. Persons who do not obtain an evaluation but who sign a release/waiver may be permitted to participate.* However, they should be encouraged to participate in only moderate- or lower-intensity physical activities and counseled about warning symptoms and signs of an impending cardiovascular event.

The major objectives of preparticipation cardiovascular screening are to identify persons with known cardiovascular disease, symptoms of cardiovascular disease, and/or risk factors for disease development who should receive a medical evaluation/recommendation before starting an exercise program or undergoing exercise testing. Screening also identifies persons with known cardiovascular disease who should not participate in an exercise program or who should participate at least initially in a medically supervised program, as well as persons with other special needs (8,19).

Screening also serves another purpose. One of the trends in cardiac rehabilitation is to "mainstream" low-risk, clinically stable patients to community facilities rather than specialized, often costly cardiac programs. Facility directors should expect that an increasing percentage of their participants will have health histories that warrant supervision of exercise programs by professional staff.

When a medical evaluation/recommendation is advised or required, written and active communication with the individual's personal physician (or healthcare provider) is strongly recommended. The sample letter and medical release form in Table 3, A and B, can be used or modified for such purposes.

TABLE 3A   Sample Physician Referral Form[a]

Dear Dr.

Your patient *(name of patient)* would like to begin a program of exercise and/or sports activity at *(name of health/fitness facility)*. After reviewing his/her responses to our cardiovascular screening questionnaire, we would appreciate your medical opinion and recommendations concerning his/her participation in exercise/ sports activity. *Please provide the following information and return this form to (name, address, telephone, fax of health/fitness facility contact):*

1. Are there specific concerns or conditions our staff should be aware of before this individual engages in exercise/sports activity at our facility? Yes/No. If yes, please specify:

   _____

   _____

2. If this individual has completed an exercise test, please provide the following:
   a. Date of test
   b. A copy of the final exercise test report and interpretation
   c. Your specific recommendations for exercise training, including heart rate limits during exercise:

   _____

   _____

3. Please provide the following information so that we may contact you if we have any further questions:
   _____ I AGREE to the participation of this individual in exercise/sports activity at your health/fitness facility.
   _____ I DO NOT AGREE that this individual is a candidate to exercise at your health/fitness facility because

   _____

   _____

Physician's signature _____

Address _____

Telephone _____   Fax _____

Thank you for your help.

---

[a] Must be accompanied by a medical release form.

TABLE 3B   Sample Authorization for Release of Medical Information

1. I hereby authorize _____ to release the following information from the medical record of

   Patient's name _____

   Address _____

   Telephone _____

   Date of birth _____

2. Information to be released: *(If specific treatment dates are not indicated, information from the most recent visit will be released.)*

   ___ Exercise test   ___ Most recent history and physical exam

   ___ Most recent clinic visit   ___ Consultations

   ___ Laboratory results (specify) _____

   ___ Other (specify) _____

3. Information to be released to:

   Name of person/organization _____

   Address _____

   Telephone _____

4. Purpose of disclosure information: _____

5. I do not give permission for disclosure or redisclosure of this information other than that specified above.

6. I request that this consent become invalid 90 days from the date I sign it or _____

I understand that this consent can be revoked at any time except to the extent that disclosure made in good faith has already occurred in reliance on this consent.

7. Patient's signature _____

   Date _____

   Witness (please print) _____

   Signature _____

Characteristics of Participants

Intensity of physical activity is measured through endurance- or strength-type exercise as defined in Table 4. Health appraisal questionnaires should be used before exercise testing and/or training to initially classify participants by risk for triage and preliminary decision making (Table 5), namely, apparently healthy persons (Class A-1), persons at increased risk (Classes A-2 and A-3), and persons with known cardiovascular disease (Classes B, C, and D). Apparently healthy persons of all ages and asymptomatic persons at increased risk (Classes A-1 through A-3) may participate in *moderate-intensity* exercise without first undergoing a medical examination or a medically supervised, symptom-limited exercise test. Apparently healthy younger persons (Class A-1) may also participate in *vigorous* exercise without first undergoing a medical examination and a medically supervised exercise test. It is suggested that persons classified as Class A-2 and particularly Class A-3 undergo a medical examination and possibly a maximal exercise test before engaging in vigorous exercise. All other persons (Classes B and C) should undergo a medical examination and perform a maximal exercise test before participation in moderate or vigorous exercise unless exercise is contraindicated (i.e., Class D). Data from a medical evaluation performed within 1 yr are acceptable unless clinical status has changed. Medically supervised exercise tests should be conducted in accordance with previously published guidelines (8).

Using Screening Results for Risk Stratification

With completion of the initial health appraisal and, if indicated, medical consultation and supervised exercise test, participants can be further classified for exercise training on the basis of individual characteristics detailed below. The following classifications have been modified using existing AHA (8) and ACSM (2) guidelines and are recommended (Table 5):

- *Class A: Apparently healthy.* There is no evidence of increased cardiovascular risk for exercise. This classification includes 1) "apparently healthy" younger persons (Class A-1) and 2) irrespective of age, persons who are "apparently healthy" or at "increased risk" (Classes A-2 and A-3) and who have a normal diagnostic maximal exercise test. Submaximal exercise tests are sometimes performed at health/fitness facilities where permitted by law for nondiagnostic purposes, including physical fitness assessment, exercise prescription, and monitoring of progress (2). Such testing is also useful for educating participants about exercise and for motivating them. Nondiagnostic exercise testing should be conducted only for persons in Class A and only by appropriately qualified, well-trained personnel (see section on staffing below) who are knowledgeable about indications and contraindications for exercise testing, indications for test termination, and test interpretation. All health/fitness facilities, including those where exercise testing is performed, should have an emergency plan (see section on emergency policies and procedures below) to ensure that emergencies are handled safely, efficiently, and effectively. No restrictions other than provision of basic guidelines are required for exercise training. No special supervision is required during exercise training.

TABLE 4 Classification of Physical Activity Intensity

	RELATIVE INTENSITY		ABSOLUTE INTENSITY RANGES (METS) ACROSS FITNESS LEVELS			
Intensity	$\dot{V}O_2R$ (%) HRR (%)	Maximal heart rate (%)	12 MET $\dot{V}O_2$max	10 MET $\dot{V}O_2$max	8 MET $\dot{V}O_2$max	6 MET $\dot{V}O_2$max
Very light	<20	<50	<3.2	<2.8	<2.4	<2.0
Light	20–39	50–63	3.2–5.3	2.8–4.5	2.4–3.7	2.0–3.0
Moderate	40–59	64–76	5.4–7.5	4.6–6.3	3.8–5.1	3.1–4.0
Hard (vigorous)	60–84	77–93	7.6–10.2	6.4–8.6	5.2–6.9	4.1–5.2
Very hard	≥85	≥94	≥10.3	≥8.7	≥7.0	≥5.3
Maximal	100	100	12.0	10.0	8.0	6.0

METs, metabolic equivalent units (1 MET = 3.5 mL · kg^{-1} · min^{-1}); oxygen uptake reserve; HRR, heart rate reserve.

Reproduced with permission from *AHA/ACSM Scientific Statement: Recommendations for Cardiovascular Screening, Staffing, and Emergency Policies at Health/Fitness Facilities* © 1998, American Heart Association.

TABLE 5 Participant/Health-Fitness Facility Selection Chart

Participant characteristics	Risk class A-1	Risk class A-2	Risk class A-3	Risk class B	Risk class C	Risk class D
Age/gender	Children	Men >45 yr	Men >45 yr	Children[a]	Children[a]	Children[a]
	Adolescents	Women >55 yr	Women >55 yr	Adolescents[a]	Adolescents[a]	Adolescents[a]
	Men <45 yr			Men	Men	Men
	Women <55 yr			Women	Women	Women
Cardiovascular risk factors	None	None	>2	May be present	May be present	May be present
Known CVD	None	None	None	Yes	Yes	Yes
CVD features (see text for details)	Class A apparently healthy	Class A apparently healthy	Class A apparently healthy	Class B known CVD: low risk	Class C known CVD: moderate risk	Class D known CVD: high risk
Low intensity	Facility 1-4	Facility 1-4	Facility 1-4	Facility 1-5	Facility 4-5	Not recommended
Moderate intensity	Facility 1-4	Facility 1-4	Facility 1-4	Facility 4-5	Facility 5	Not recommended
Vigorous intensity	Facility 1-4	Facility 1-4	Facility 1-4	Facility 4-5	Facility 5	Not recommended

	FACILITY CHARACTERISTICS				
	Level 1	Level 2	Level 3	Level 4	Level 6
Type of facility	Unsupervised exercise room	Single exercise leader	Fitness center for healthy clients	Fitness center serving clinical populations	Medically supervised clinical exercise program
Personnel	None	• Exercise leader • Recommended: medical liaison	• General manager • Health/fitness instructor • Exercise leader • Recommended: medical liaison	• General manager • Exercise specialist • Health/fitness instructor • Medical liaison	• General manager • Exercise specialist • Health/fitness instructor • Medical liaison
Emergency plan	Present	Present	Present	Present	Present
Emergency equipment	• Telephone in room • Signs	• Telephone • Signs • Recommended: blood pressure kit; stethoscope	• Telephone • Signs • Recommended: blood pressure kit; stethoscope	• Telephone • Signs • Blood pressure kit • Stethoscope	• Telephone • Signs • Blood pressure kit • Stethoscope • Oxygen • Crash cart • Defibrillator

[a] Risk stratification for patients with congenital heart disease should be guided by recommendations of the 26th Bethesda Conference (28). CVD indicates cardiovascular disease.

• *Class B: Presence of known, stable cardiovascular disease with low risk for vigorous exercise but slightly greater than for apparently healthy persons.* This classification includes clinically stable persons with 1) coronary artery disease (myocardial infarction, coronary artery bypass surgery, percutaneous transluminal coronary angioplasty, angina pectoris, abnormal exercise test, or abnormal coronary angiogram); 2) valvular heart disease; 3) congenital heart disease (risk stratification for patients with congenital heart disease should be guided by the 26th Bethesda Conference recommendations (28)); 4) cardiomyopathy (includes stable patients with heart failure with characteristics as outlined below but not recent myocarditis or hypertrophic cardiomyopathy); and 5) exercise test abnormalities that do not meet the criteria outlined in Class C below. The clinical characteristics of such persons are 1) New York Heart Association (NYHA) Class I or II (Table 6); 2) exercise capacity >6 METs; 3) no evidence of heart failure; 4) free of ischemia or angina at rest or on the exercise test ≤ 6 METs; 5) appropriate rise in systolic blood pressure during exercise; 6) absence of nonsustained or sustained ventricular tachycardia; and 7) ability to satisfactorily self-monitor intensity of activity. For these persons, activity should be individualized with exercise prescription by qualified personnel. Medical supervision is recommended during prescription sessions and nonmedical supervision by appropriately qualified staff for other exercise sessions until the participant understands how to monitor his or her own activity. Subsequent exercise training may be performed without special supervision.

• *Class C: Those at moderate to high risk for cardiac complications during exercise and/or who are unable to self-regulate activity or understand the recommended activity level.* This classification includes persons with 1) coronary artery disease with the clinical characteristics outlined below; 2) acquired valvular heart disease; 3) congenital heart disease (risk stratification for patients with congenital heart disease should be guided by the 26th Bethesda Conference recommendations (28)); 4) cardiomyopathy (includes stable patients with heart failure with characteristics as outlined below but not recent myocarditis or hypertrophic cardiomyopathy); 5) exercise test abnormalities not directly related to ischemia; 6) a previous episode of ventricular fibrillation or cardiac arrest that did not occur in the presence of an acute ischemic event or cardiac procedure; 7) complex ventricular arrhythmias that are uncontrolled at mild to moderate work intensity with medication; 8) three-vessel or left main coronary artery disease; and 9) ejection fraction < 30%. One or more of the following clinical characteristics are also present: 1) two or more previous myocardial infarctions; 2) NYHA Class III or greater; 3) exercise capacity < 6 METs; 4) ischemic horizontal or down-sloping ST depression ≥ 1 mm or angina at a workload ≤ 6 METs; 5) a fall in systolic blood pressure with exercise; 6) a medical problem that the physician believes may be potentially life-threatening; 7) a previous episode of primary cardiac arrest; and 8) ventricular tachycardia at a workload < 6 METs. Physical activity should be individualized, and exercise should be prescribed by appropriately qualified medical personnel. Medical supervision, monitoring for adverse signs and symptoms, electrocardiographic monitoring of heart rate and rhythm, and blood pressure monitoring are recommended during exercise sessions until safety is established. Subsequent exercise training should be supervised by appropriately qualified personnel.

• *Class D: Unstable conditions with activity restriction.* This classification includes those with 1) unstable ischemia; 2) heart failure that is not compensated; 3) uncontrolled arrhythmias; 4) severe and symptomatic aortic stenosis; 5) hypertrophic cardiomyopathy or cardiomyopathy from recent myocarditis; 6) severe pulmonary hypertension; or 7) other conditions that could be aggravated by exercise (for example, resting systolic blood pressure >200 mm Hg or resting diastolic blood pressure >110 mm Hg; active or suspected myocarditis or pericarditis; suspected or known dissecting aneurysm; thrombophlebitis and recent systemic or pulmonary embolus). In this population no physical activity is recommended for conditioning purposes. Risk stratification for patients with congenital heart disease should be guided by the 26th Bethesda Conference recommendations (28).

TABLE 6	New York Heart Association Classification (8)
Class I	Heart disease without symptoms
Class II	Heart disease with symptoms during ordinary activity
Class III	Heart disease with symptoms during less than ordinary activity
Class IV	Heart disease with symptoms at rest

These classifications are presented as a means of beginning exercise with the lowest possible risk. They do not consider accompanying morbidities (for example, insulin-dependent diabetes mellitus, morbid obesity, severe pulmonary disease, complicated pregnancy, or debilitating neurological or orthopedic conditions) that may constitute a contraindication to exercise or necessitate closer supervision during exercise training.

Using Screening Results for Exercise Prescription

For individuals considered to be in Class A, exercise training intensity (Table 4) may be prescribed using the rating of perceived exertion alone and/or specific target heart rates. A suggested rating of perceived exertion for such persons is 12-16 (moderate to hard) on the Borg scale of 6-20 and/or an intensity level that corresponds to 50-90% of maximum heart rate or 45-85% of maximum oxygen uptake or heart rate reserve. Heart rate reserve is defined as maximum heart rate minus resting heart rate. For persons taking medications that affect heart rate (e.g., beta-adrenergic blockers), these heart rate methods do not apply unless guided by an exercise tolerance test.

In the absence of atrial fibrillation, frequent atrial or ventricular ectopy, a fixed-rate pacemaker, or similar conditions, exercise intensity should be prescribed for persons with cardiovascular disease (Class B or C) using target heart rates and perceived exertion ratings in accordance with previously published guidelines (2,8). For these persons, target heart rates should be prescribed using data obtained during exercise testing performed while the participant is taking his or her usual cardioactive medications. In the absence of myocardial ischemia or other significant exercise test abnormalities, a target range of 50-90% of peak heart rate or 45-85% of peak measured oxygen uptake or heart rate reserve is recommended. This intensity level corresponds to 12-16 (moderate to hard) on the Borg scale. In the presence of myocardial ischemia (i.e., ischemic ST-segment depression >1 mm, chest discomfort believed to be angina pectoris, or other symptoms believed to be an anginal equivalent), significant arrhythmia, or other significant exercise test abnormalities (e.g., a fall in systolic blood pressure from baseline, systolic blood pressure >240 mm Hg, or diastolic blood pressure >110 mm Hg), the target training intensity is derived from the heart rate associated with the abnormality. If this occurs at a high level of exercise, the above target heart rate recommendations are applicable, provided that the upper limit of the range is at least 10 beats per minute (bpm) below the level at which the abnormality appears. Otherwise, the recommended upper limit of train-ing heart rate is 10 bpm less than that associated with the abnormality.

STAFFING

Health/fitness facility personnel involved in management or delivery of exercise programs must meet academic and professional standards and have the required experience as established by the ACSM (2,19). Such personnel include the general manager/executive director, medical liaison, fitness director, and exercise leader. In general, health/fitness facility personnel should have the formal training and experience needed to ensure that clients are provided with safe, effective programs and services. The levels of education and experience needed to ensure effectiveness and safety vary with the health status of the client population. The kinds of personnel who should be employed at health/fitness facilities serving various types of clients are summarized in Table 5.

The general manager/executive director is responsible for the overall management of the facility and should have competencies in business as well as design and delivery of exercise programs.

The medical liaison reviews medical emergency plans, witnesses and critiques medical emergency drills, and reviews medical incident reports. In level 2 and 3 facilities (Table 5), the medical liaison may be a licensed physician, a registered nurse trained in advanced cardiac life support, or an emergency medical technician. In level 4 and 5 facilities (Table 5), the medical liaison must be a licensed physician.

The fitness director manages the facility's exercise and activity programs and is responsible for program design and the training and supervision of staff. He or she must have a degree in exercise science, another health-related field, or equivalent experience, and knowledge of exercise physiology, exercise programming, and operation of exercise facilities. The fitness director must hold professional certification at an advanced level by a nationally recognized health/fitness organization. In level 3 facilities this certification should be comparable to ACSM health fitness instructor certification. In level 4 and 5 facilities the fitness director should be certified at a level that correlates with ACSM exercise specialist certification. The exercise specialist typically holds a master's degree in exercise science or a related field and has extensive experience in exercise testing and leadership in clinical populations. He or she must be trained in cardiopulmonary resuscitation (CPR) and should have at least 1 yr of supervisory experience in the fitness industry.

The exercise leader works directly with program participants and provides instruction and leadership in specific modes of exercise. He or she also helps program participants master the behavioral skills needed to adhere to exercise programs. In level 1, 2, and 3 facilities the exercise leader as a minimum must have a high school diploma or equivalent and entry-level or higher professional certification from a nationally recognized health/fitness organization (comparable to ACSM exercise leader certification). In level 4 facilities, the exercise leader should have education and experience corresponding to that required by ACSM health fitness instructor certification. In level 5 facilities, the exercise leader should be either an exercise specialist or a health fitness instructor directly supervised by an exercise specialist. *In all cases the exercise leader must be trained in CPR and should have prior supervised internship or work experience in the health/fitness industry.*

Some health/fitness facilities provide services in allied health fields such as nutrition, stress management, and physical therapy. Personnel providing such services should meet current accepted professional standards in those fields and should be certified as recommended by relevant professional organizations and licensed by or registered with the state as required by law.

EMERGENCY POLICIES AND PROCEDURES

All health/fitness facilities must have written emergency policies and procedures that are reviewed and practiced regularly. Such plans will correspond to the type of facility and risk level of its membership outlined in Table 5. All fitness center staff who directly supervise program participants should be trained in basic life support. Health/fitness facilities must develop appropriate emergency response plans and must train their staff in appropriate procedures to provide during a life-threatening emergency. When an incident occurs, each staff member must perform the necessary emergency support steps in accordance with established procedures. It is important for everyone to know the emergency plan. Emergency drills should be practiced once every 3 months or more often with changes in staff; retraining and rehearsal are especially important. When new staff are hired, new team arrangements may be necessary. Because life-threatening cardiovascular emergencies are rare, constant vigilance by staff and familiarity with the plan and how to follow it are important.

It is essential to acknowledge that emergency equipment alone does not save lives. Equipment alone may offer a false sense of security if it is not backed up with appropriate staffing. The training and preparedness of an astute professional staff who can readily handle emergencies is paramount. This issue is particularly important if persons with certain medical conditions are recruited and encouraged to exercise in a specific health/fitness facility. Such a facility has the responsibility to offer appropriate coverage by personnel as outlined above and in Table 5. Acquisition of equipment for evaluation and resuscitation will depend on the risk level of participants, personnel, and medical coverage. All facilities must have a telephone that is readily accessible and available when emergency assistance is needed. It would be useful for all supervised facilities to have a sphygmomanometer and stethoscope readily available. Level 4 and 5 facilities that recruit members with known cardiovascular disease must have such equipment available, and level 5 (supervised cardiac rehabilitation) facilities should be fully equipped according to the recommendations of the AHA (21) and the American Association of Cardiovascular and Pulmonary Rehabilitation (1). Such equipment includes a defibrillator, oxygen, and fully stocked crash cart. Delineation of specific equipment standards in such facilities is beyond the scope of these guidelines; such information is detailed in the documents above (1,21). Appropriately trained staff who are medically and legally empowered must be available to operate such devices during a facility's operational hours.

The emergency plan must address transportation of victims to a hospital emergency room and must include telephone access to 911 or the local emergency unit access system. Health/fitness facility personnel should be familiar with emergency transport teams in the area so that access and location of the center are clearly identified. Staff should greet the emergency response team at the entrance of the facility so that they can be promptly guided to the site of the emergency. A staff member should remain with the victim at all times. Prompt emergency transport is optimized by free and ready access to the victim within the health/fitness facility and assistance by designated staff.

GENERAL CONSIDERATIONS IN SELECTING A HEALTH/FITNESS FACILITY

In selecting a health/fitness facility, an individual should first consider his or her health status. Persons with a history of cardiovascular disease should seek facilities that provide or require a thorough medical evaluation of prospective members/users. Personnel should include nurses, exercise specialists, health/fitness instructors, and/or exercise leaders licensed or certified by the appropriate agencies, organizations, or authorities. They should be trained to recommend and supervise exercise in patients with cardiovascular and other chronic diseases. Persons at high risk for development of cardiovascular disease should seek facilities that require appropriate medical evaluation of clients and employ exercise leaders who are certified as competent to design and deliver exercise programs for high-risk persons. Table 5 summarizes personnel and safety recommendations for health/fitness facilities (levels 1 through 5) serving clients in various health categories (Classes A through C).

Persons seeking health/fitness facilities should select one that meets professional and industry standards. Facilities should be clean, well-maintained, and spacious enough to ensure the comfort and safety of program participants. Indoor facilities should be climate controlled, and changing rooms and showers should be provided. Flooring in areas where exercise is to be carried out should be designed to minimize risk of injury. Exercise equipment should be well-maintained. The variety, amount, and availability of exercise equipment should match individual needs and preferences, including time of day and preferred mode of exercise. For example, if aerobic dance is the preferred mode of exercise, individuals should seek a fitness center that offers this program at a convenient time and that provides an exercise leader who is competent in this activity and able to teach men and women of various age and fitness levels.

The programs and services of a health/fitness center should optimize participation. The location of the center should minimize time spent traveling to it. The social environment should be attractive and the staff competent in helping members/users master the behavioral skills needed to adopt and maintain a physically active lifestyle.

SUMMARY OF KEY POINTS

- Physical inactivity is a risk factor for cardiovascular disease; it is very prevalent and an important health issue.
- Regular exercise reduces subsequent cardiovascular morbidity and mortality (7,17,18).

- Efforts to promote physical activity will impact everyone, including persons with cardiovascular disease.
- The incidence of a cardiovascular event during exercise among patients with cardiac disease is greater than that among otherwise healthy persons (8).
- Overall, in the general population the absolute incidence of death during exercise is relatively low (8).
- *All facilities offering exercise equipment or services should conduct a cardiovascular screening of all new members and/or prospective users.* Preparticipation screening should identify persons at high risk, and public health efforts should focus on increasing the use of screening. In view of the potential legal risk assumed by operators of fitness facilities, it is recommended that those facilities providing staff supervision document the results of screening.
- When a medical evaluation/recommendation is advised or required, written and active communication by facility staff with the individual's personal physician (or healthcare provider) is strongly recommended.
- Health appraisal questionnaires should be used before exercise testing and/or training to initially classify participants by risk for triage and preliminary decision making. After the initial health appraisal and, if indicated, medical consultation and supervised exercise test, participants can be further classified for exercise training on the basis of individual characteristics.
- Every effort should be made to educate participants about the importance of obtaining a preparticipation health appraisal and, if indicated, a medical evaluation/recommendation. The potential risks incurred without obtaining an appraisal and/or evaluation should also be emphasized.
- *The AHA, the IHRSA, and the ACSM recommend that all health/fitness facilities have written emergency policies and procedures that are reviewed and practiced regularly (16,19).* It is essential to acknowledge that emergency equipment alone does not save lives: training and preparedness by astute professional staff who can readily handle emergencies is paramount.
- Whatever their health status, persons seeking a health/fitness facility should choose one that provides equipment, programs, staff, services,

and membership contracts appropriate for their needs and that meets accepted professional and industry standards.

REFERENCES

1. American Association of Cardiovascular, and Pulmonary Rehabilitation. *Guidelines for Cardiac Rehabilitation Programs,* 2nd Ed. Champaign, IL: Human Kinetics Publishers, 1995.

2. American College of Sports Medicine. *Guidelines for Exercise Testing and Prescription,* 5th Ed., W.L. Kenney (Ed.). Baltimore: Williams & Wilkins, 1995:269-287.

3. American Heart Association. *Heart and Stroke Facts: 1997 Statistical Supplement.* Dallas: AHA, 1996.

4. Anderson, K.M., P.W. Wilson, P.M. Odell, and W.B. Kannel. An updated coronary risk profile: a statement for health professionals. *Circulation* 83:356-362, 1991.

5. Borg, G.A. Psychophysical basis of perceived exertion. *Med. Sci. Sports Exerc.* 14:377-381, 1982.

6. Fletcher, G. How to implement physical activity in primary and secondary prevention: a statement for healthcare professionals from the American Heart Association. *Circulation* 96:355-357, 1997.

7. Fletcher, G.F., G.J. Balady, S.N. Blair, et al. Statement on exercise: benefits and recommendations for physical activity programs for all Americans. *Circulation* 94:857-862, 1996.

8. Fletcher, G.F., G.J. Balady, V.F. Froelicher, L.H. Hartley, W.L. Haskell, and M.L. Pollock. Exercise standards: a statement from the American Heart Association. *Circulation* 91:580-615, 1995.

9. Gibbons, R.J., G.J. Balady, J.W. Beasley, et al. ACC/AHA guidelines for exercise testing: a report of the American College of Cardiology/American Heart Association Task Force on Practice Guidelines. *J. Am. Coll. Cardiol.* 30:260-311, 1997.

10. Healthy People 2000: National Health Promotion and Disease Prevention Objectives. U.S. Dept. of Health and Human Services/Public Health Service. Publication no. (PHS) 91-50213.

11. *How to Choose a Health Club.* Milwaukee, WI: Wisconsin Affiliate, American Heart Association, 1989.

12. Maron, B.J., P.D. Thompson, J.C. Puffer, et al. Cardiovascular preparticipation screening of competitive athletes: a statement for health professionals from the American Heart Association. *Circulation* 94:850-856, 1996.

13. Maron, B.J., J. Shirani, L.C. Poliac, R. Mathenge, W.C. Roberts, and F.O. Mueller. Sudden death in young competitive athletes: clinical, demographic, and pathological profiles. *J.A.M.A.* 276:199-204, 1996.

14. McInnis, K.J., S. Hayakawa, and G.J. Balady. Cardiovascular screening and emergency procedures at health clubs and fitness centers. *Am. J. Cardiol.* 80:380-383, 1997.

15. Mittleman, M.A., M. Maclure, G.H. Tofler, J.B. Sherwood, R.J. Goldberg, and J.E. Muller. Triggering of acute myocardial infarction by heavy physical exertion: protection against triggering by regular exertion. *N. Engl. J. Med.* 329:1677-1683, 1993.

16. *1997 IHRSA/American Sports Data Health Club Trend Report.* Hartsdale, NY: American Sports Data, 1997.

17. Paffenbarger, R.S., R.T. Hyde, A.L. Wing, and C.C. Hsieh. Physical activity, all-cause mortality, and longevity of college alumni. *N. Engl. J. Med.* 314:605-613, 1986.

18. Pate, R.R., M. Pratt, S.N. Blair, et al. Physical activity and public health: a recommendation from the Centers for Disease Control and Prevention and the American College of Sports Medicine. *J.A.M.A.* 273:402-407, 1995.

19. Peterson, J.A., and S.J. Tharrett, eds. *American College of Sports Medicine Health/Fitness Facility Standards and Guidelines,* 2nd Ed. Champaign, IL: Human Kinetics Publishers, 1997.

20. *Physical Activity and Health: A Report of the Surgeon General.* Atlanta: U.S. Department of Health and Human Services, Centers for Disease Control and Prevention, National Center for Chronic Disease Prevention and Health Promotion, 1996.

21. Pina, I.L., G.J. Balady, P. Hanson, A.J. Labovitz, D.W. Madonna, and J. Myers. Guidelines for clinical exercise testing laboratories: a statement for healthcare professionals from the American Heart Association. *Circulation* 91:912-921, 1995.

22. Shephard, R.J., S. Thomas, and I. Weller. The Canadian home fitness test: 1991 update. *Sports Med.* 11:358-366, 1991.

23. Siscovick, D.S., N.S. Weiss, R.H. Fletcher, and T. Lasky. The incidence of primary cardiac arrest during vigorous exercise. *N. Engl. J. Med.* 311:874-877, 1984.

24. Thomas, S., J. Reading, and R.J. Shephard. Revision of the Physical Activity Readiness Questionnaire (PAR-Q). *Can. J. Sports Sci.* 17:338-345, 1992.

25. Thompson, P.D. The cardiovascular complications of vigorous physical activity. *Arch. Intern. Med.* 156:2297-2302, 1996.

26. Thompson, P.D., E.J. Funk, R.A. Carleton, and W.Q. Sturner. Incidence of death during jogging in Rhode Island from 1975 through 1980. *J.A.M.A.* 247:2535-2538, 1982.

27. Tofler, G.H., J.E. Muller, P.H. Stone, et al. Modifiers of timing and possible triggers of acute myocardial infarction in the Thrombolysis in Myocardial Infarction Phase II (TIMI II) study group. *J. Am. Coll. Cardiol.* 20:1049-1055, 1992.

28. 26th Bethesda Conference. Recommendations for determining eligibility for competition in athletes with cardiovascular abnormalities. *J. Am. Coll. Cardiol.* 24:845-899, 1994.

29. Van Camp, S.P., C.M. Bloor, F.O. Mueller, R.C. Cantu, and H.G. Olson. Nontraumatic sports death in high school and college athletes. *Med. Sci. Sports Exerc.* 27:641-647, 1995.

30. Van Camp, S.P., and R.A. Peterson. Cardiovascular complications of outpatient cardiac rehabilitation programs. *J.A.M.A.* 256:1160-1163, 1986.

31. Willich, S.N., M. Lewis, II. Lowel, H.R. Arntz, F. Schubert, and R. Schroder. Physical exertion as a trigger of acute myocardial infarction. *N. Engl. J. Med.* 329:1684-1690, 1993.

This scientific statement was written by Gary J. Balady, M.D., Chair; Bernard Chaitman, M.D.; David Driscoll, M.D.; Carl Foster, Ph.D.; Erika Froelicher, Ph.D.; Neil Gordon, M.D.; Russell Pate, Ph.D.; James Rippe, M.D.; and Terry Bazzarre, Ph.D.

ACSM/AHA Joint Position Statement

Automated External Defibrillators in Health/Fitness Facilities

In 1998, the AHA/ACSM published recommendations (5,6) for health/fitness facilities regarding the screening of clients for the presence of cardiovascular disease, appropriate staffing, emergency policies, equipment, and procedures relative to the client base of a given facility. Accordingly, health/fitness facilities are defined as organizations that offer exercise-based health and fitness programs as their primary or secondary service or that promote moderate- to vigorous-intensity recreational physical activity. These range from level 1 (unsupervised exercise room) to level 5 (medically supervised exercise program), and their specific characteristics are outlined in Table 1. Details regarding emergency readiness are provided in the AHA/ACSM recommendations (5,6) and emphasize that all health/fitness facilities must have written emergency policies and procedures that are reviewed and practiced regularly, and that in all supervised facilities, exercise leaders must be trained in basic cardiopulmonary resuscitation (CPR). Because of

the publication of the 1998 AHA/ACSM recommendations, 47 states have since passed Good Samaritan legislation, and the federal government has passed the Cardiac Arrest Survival Act and the Rural Access to Emergency Devices Act as components of the federal Public Health Improvement Act of 2000 (7). These state and federal laws now serve to expand Good Samaritan legal protections to users of automated external defibrillators (AEDs) throughout the nation. Therefore, the purpose of this statement is to supplement the 1998 AHA/ACSM recommendations (5,6) regarding the purchase and use of AEDs in health/fitness facilities. Similar to the parent document (5,6), these recommendations are based on a review of the literature and consensus of the writing group after having undergone extensive peer review and final approval by AHA and ACSM. The recommendations are not mandatory or all encompassing, nor do they limit provision of individualized care by health/fitness facilities exercising independent judgment.

This joint position paper was authored by the American College of Sports Medicine and the American Heart Association, and the content appears in AHA style. This paper is being published concurrently in *Medicine & Science in Sports & Exercise* and in *Circulation*. Individual name recognition is reflected in the acknowledgements at the end of the statement.

TABLE 1	Health/Fitness Facilities Emergency Plans and Equipment[a]				
	Level 1	**Level 2**	**Level 3**	**Level 4**	**Level 5**
Type of facility	Unsupervised exercise room (e.g., those in hotels, commercial buildings, and apartment complexes)	Single exercise leader	Fitness center for general membership	Fitness center offering special programs for clinical populations	Medically supervised clinical exercise program (e.g., cardiac rehabilitation)
Personnel[b]	None	• Exercise leader • Recommended: medical liaison	• General manager • Health/fitness instructor • Exercise leader • Recommended: medical liaison	• General manager • Exercise specialist • Health/fitness instructor • Medical liaison	• General manager • Exercise specialist • Health/fitness instructor • Medical liaison
Emergency plan	Present	Present	Present	Present	Present
Emergency equipment	• Telephone in room • Signs • Encouraged: PAD plan with AED as part of the composite PAD plan in the host facility (e.g., hotel, commercial building, apartment complex)	• Telephone • Signs • Encouraged: blood pressure kit, stethoscope, PAD plan with AED	• Telephone • Signs • Encouraged: blood pressure kit, stethoscope, PAD plan with AED (the latter are strongly encouraged in facilities with membership >2,500 and those in which EMS response time is expected to be >5 min from recognition of arrest)	• Telephone • Signs • Blood pressure kit • Stethoscope • Strongly encouraged: PAD plan with AED	• Telephone • Signs • Blood pressure kit • Stethoscope • Oxygen • Crash cart • Defibrillator[c]

AED, automatic external defibrillator; PAD, public access to defibrillator.

[a] This table should replace the bottom half of Table 5 of the AHA/ACSM Recommendations (5,6).

[b] Detailed definitions and competencies for personnel positions are outlined in the ACSM Guidelines (10).

[c] Standard equipment in level 5 facilities includes a defibrillator (5,6,22).

ROLE OF AEDS IN THE CHAIN OF SURVIVAL

An AED is a device that incorporates a rhythm-analysis system and a shock-advisory system for victims of cardiac arrest (1). The AED advises a shock, and the operator must take the final action to deliver the shock. The International Guidelines for Cardiopulmonary Resuscitation and Emergency Cardiovascular Care (2) conclude that early CPR is the best treatment for cardiac arrest until the arrival of an AED and advanced cardiac life support care. The chain of survival includes a series of actions designed to reduce mortality associated with cardiac arrest. Early CPR plays an important role in the chain of survival that includes the following links:

1) early recognition of cardiopulmonary arrest, 2) early CPR, 3) early defibrillation when indicated, and 4) early advanced cardiac life support care (3). Early CPR can prevent ventricular fibrillation from deteriorating to asystole, may increase the chance of successful defibrillation, contributes to the preservation of heart and brain function, and significantly improves survival (4). Importantly, for victims of sudden, shockable cardiac arrest (ventricular fibrillation or pulseless ventricular tachycardia), the single greatest determinant of survival is the time from collapse to defibrillation. A recent review (17) summarizes the data comparing the time-to-shock between first responders (i.e., firefighters, police, and emergency medical system (EMS) basic life support personnel) versus paramedics and demon-

strates significantly shorter times among first responders in three of five studies. A survival rate, among victims of witnessed ventricular fibrillation cardiac arrest, as high as 90% has been reported when defibrillation is achieved within the first minute of collapse (8,11,14,15,21). Survival rates decline 7-10% with every minute that defibrillation is delayed, such that a cardiac arrest victim without defibrillation beyond 12 minutes has only a 2-5% chance of survival (1). The highest survival rates for out of hospital cardiac arrest have been reported in cardiac rehabilitation programs equipped with defibrillators (i.e., Table 1: level-5 facilities), where survival approaches 90% (8,11,14,15,21). The International Guidelines (2) conclude that public access to defibrillation (PAD) accomplished by the placement of AEDs in selected locations for immediate use by trained laypersons may be the key intervention to significantly increase survival from an out-of-hospital cardiac arrest. Two recent observational studies report impressive results regarding the effectiveness of PAD in persons with witnessed cardiac arrest, who are in ventricular fibrillation, with AED placement in casinos (20) and on airplanes (19). The cardiac arrest survival rates to discharge from the hospital were 53% and 40%, respectively.

CARDIOVASCULAR RISKS OF EXERCISE

The AHA/ACSM Recommendations (5,6) provide details regarding the cardiovascular risks of exercise. It is clear that the risk of adverse cardiovascular events including death is greater among those individuals with cardiovascular disease than among presumably healthy individuals (5,6,9). As the demographics of the more than 30 million individuals who exercise at health/fitness facilities demonstrate a steady increase in the number of members older than 35 yr (approximately 55% of current membership) (16), it is reasonable to presume that the number of members with cardiovascular disease (and other comorbidities) is rising as well. Although there are no data regarding the incidence of cardiac arrest at health/fitness facilities, two recent surveys provide some important insight. A large database consisting of more than 2.9 million members of a large commercial health/fitness facility chain demonstrates 71 deaths (mean age 52 ± 13 yr; 61 men, 10 women) occurring over a 2-year period, yielding a rate of 1 death/100,000 members/year. The death rate was highest among those members who exercised less

frequently, such that nearly half of exercise-related deaths were in those who exercised less than once/ week (12). The cardiac arrest rate was not reported but was presumably higher than the death rate. A recent survey of 65 randomly chosen health/fitness facilities in Ohio (18) reports the occurrence of sudden cardiac arrest or heart attack in 17% of facilities during a 5-year period. Notably, only 3% of facilities had an AED on site. Thus, it is prudent to conclude that health/fitness facilities should be considered among the sites in which PAD programs should be established.

RECOMMENDATIONS

It is essential to acknowledge that emergency equipment alone does not save lives. The ACSM/AHA Recommendations (5,6) emphasize the importance of written emergency policies and procedures that are reviewed and practiced regularly. Well-trained health/fitness facility staff members are essential to maintain strong links in the chain of survival for their clients. Effective placement and use of AEDs at all health/fitness facilities (Table 1: levels 1-5) is encouraged, as permitted by law, to achieve the goal of minimizing the time between recognition of cardiac arrest and successful defibrillation. Until further definitive data are available, AED placement is strongly encouraged in those health/fitness facilities with a large number of members (i.e., membership > 2500; [> median size health/fitness facility (16)]); those that offer special programs to clinical populations (i.e., programs for the elderly or those with medical conditions (level 4)) (note that in level-5 facilities, current equipment standards require defibrillators (5,6,22)); and those health/fitness facilities in which the time from the recognition of cardiac arrest until the first shock is delivered by the EMS is anticipated to be > 5 minutes. In unsupervised exercise rooms (level-1 facilities), such as those that might be located in hotels, apartment complexes, or office buildings, the AED should be part of the overall PAD plan for the host facility. At the least, an unsupervised exercise room should have a telephone available in the room with clearly posted numbers to call in case of emergency. In supervised settings, it is essential that designated health/fitness facility staff members who are trained in CPR be present during all hours of operation. CPR should be initiated as soon as a cardiac arrest is recognized and should be continued until the AED is placed on the victim and is activated. In cases of cardiac arrest not due to ventricular fibrillation (VF) or pulseless ventricular tachycardia (VT), AEDs are of no value, and CPR must be maintained. Also, after successful termination of VF/pulseless VT, the rescuer must be able to open the airway and support ventilation and circulation with chest compressions as needed until the arrival of EMS personnel.

Therefore, the establishment of a PAD at all health/fitness facilities is encouraged. This plan should include the following:

- Have written emergency policies and procedures that are practiced regularly (i.e., at least once every 3 months).

- Designate staff members who are trained in CPR and function as first responders in the health/fitness facility setting during all hours of operation.

- Train staff to recognize cardiac arrest.

- Activate EMS—assign staff to meet the emergency response team at the entrance of the facility so that they can be promptly guided to the victim.

- Provide CPR.

- Attach/operate AED (detailed instructions are provided by the specific equipment manufacturer and general recommendations are outlined in the Guidelines 2000 for Cardiopulmonary Resuscitation and Emergency Cardiovascular Care (1)).

- The use of AEDs on infants and children < 8 yr of age is not recommended (1).

Health/fitness facilities should coordinate their PAD program with the local EMS, because many dispatch systems use local phone-directed protocols to assist rescuers in the use of AED and may notify local EMS en route that an AED is being used at the scene. Moreover, the local EMS may assist with program planning and quality improvement, including medical direction, AED deployment and protocols, training, monitoring, and review of AED events (1). Emergency drills should be practiced at least once every 3 months or more often when staff changes occur (5,6). When new staff are hired, new team arrangements may be necessary. The simulated use of AEDs in drills offers the best opportunity for skills maintenance. Maintaining the AED device in proper working condition according to the manufacturer's recommendations is essential. PAD programs must comply with local or regional regulation and legislation.

COSTS

Details regarding the technical aspects of AEDs are available elsewhere (1,17). At present, the cost of an AED is approximately $3000–$4500 per unit. It is expected that the price of AEDs will likely decrease as their use becomes more widespread. The National Heart Lung and Blood Institute (NHLBI), in partnership with the AHA and industry, is conducting a multisite, controlled, prospective study to determine the efficacy and cost-effectiveness of placing AEDs in a variety of public settings. A recent independent study (13) has demonstrated that a program of placing AEDs on large (> 200 passenger) and medium (> 100 passenger) capacity aircraft attain generally accepted levels of cost-effectiveness. However, the cost-effectiveness of AED deployment on smaller aircraft is, at this time, less certain. Similarly, as the cost-effectiveness of AED placement in health/fitness facilities is unknown, it is expected that these recommendations will be reviewed and updated when such data become available. At this time, individual health/fitness facilities are encouraged to maintain data on the utility of their PAD programs and perhaps engage in a collaborative effort with other health/fitness facilities to assess the success of their programs.

SUMMARY OF KEY POINTS

- The Cardiac Arrest Survival Act and the Rural Access to Emergency Devices Act, as components of the federal Public Health Improvement Act of 2000, as well as Good Samaritan laws passed in 47 states, expands Good Samaritan legal protections to users of AEDs throughout the nation.

- The placement of AEDs in selected locations for immediate use by trained laypersons may be the key intervention to significantly increase survival from an out-of-hospital cardiac arrest.

- The chain of survival includes a series of actions designed to reduce mortality associated with cardiac arrest and includes the following links: 1) early recognition of cardiopulmonary arrest, 2) early CPR, 3) early defibrillation when indicated, and 4) early advanced cardiac life support care.

- Well-trained health/fitness facility staff members are essential to maintain strong links in the chain of survival for their clients.

- Effective placement and use of AEDs at all health/fitness facilities (Table 1: levels 1-5) is encouraged, as permitted by law, to achieve the goal of minimizing the time between recognition of cardiac arrest and successful defibrillation. Until further definitive data are available, AED placement is strongly encouraged in those health/fitness facilities with a large number of members (i.e., membership > 2500); those that offer special programs to clinical populations (i.e., programs for the elderly or those with medical conditions (level 4)); and those health/fitness facilities in which the time from the recognition of cardiac arrest until the first shock is delivered by the EMS is anticipated to be > 5 minutes. In unsupervised exercise rooms (level-1 facilities), such as those that might be located in hotels, apartment complexes, or office buildings, the AED should be part of the overall PAD plan for the host facility.

- Health/fitness facilities should coordinate their PAD program with the local EMS.

- Emergency drills should be practiced at least once every 3 months or more often when staff changes occur.

- PAD programs must comply with local or regional regulation and legislation.

This work is a supplement to the AHA/ACSM Recommendations for Cardiovascular Screening, Staffing, and Emergency Policies at Health/Fitness Facilities (5,6).

Writing Group: Gary J. Balady, M.D., Chair; Bernard Chaitman, M.D.; Carl Foster, Ph.D., FACSM; Erika Froelicher, Ph.D.; Neil Gordon, M.D., FACSM; and Steven Van Camp, M.D., FACSM.

REFERENCES

1. American Heart Association and International Liaison Committee on Resuscitation. Guidelines 2000 for Cardiopulmonary Resuscitation and Emergency Cardiovascular Care. *Circulation* 102(Suppl. 1):I60–76, 2000.

2. American Heart Association and International Liaison Committee on Resuscitation. Guidelines 2000 for Cardiopulmonary Resuscitation and Emergency Cardiovascular Care. *Circulation* 102(Suppl. 1):I1–375, 2000.

3. American Heart Association and International Liaison Committee on Resuscitation. Guidelines 2000 for Cardiopulmonary Resuscitation and Emergency Cardiovascular Care. *Circulation* 102(Suppl. 1):I358–370, 2000.

4. American Heart Association and International Liaison Committee on Resuscitation. Guidelines 2000 for Cardiopulmonary Resuscitation and Emergency Cardiovascular Care. *Circulation* 102(Suppl. 1):I22–59, 2000.

5. Balady, G.J., B. Chaitman, D. Driscoll, et al. American Heart Association/American College of Sports Medicine Joint Scientific Statement: Recommendations for Cardiovascular Screening, Staffing, and Emergency Policies at Health/Fitness Facilities. *Circulation* 97:2283–2293, 1998.

6. Balady, G.J., B. Chaitman, D. Driscoll, et al. American Heart Association/American College of Sports Medicine Joint Scientific Statement: Recommendations for Cardiovascular Screening, Staffing, and Emergency Policies at Health/Fitness Facilities. *Med. Sci. Sports Exerc* 30:1009–1018, 1998.

7. Cardiac Arrest Survival Act of 2000. Public Law 106–505, Sec. 401–404.

8. Fletcher, G.F., and J.D. Cantwell. Ventricular fibrillation in a medically supervised cardiac exercise program: clinical, angiographic and surgical correlations. *JAMA* 238:2627–2629, 1977.

9. Fletcher, G.F., G.J. Balady, V.F. Froelicher, L.H. Hartley, W.H. Haskell, and M.L. Pollock. Exercise standards: a statement for health professionals from the American Heart Association. *Circulation* 91:580–615, 1995.

10. Franklin, B. (ed.). *American College of Sports Medicine Guidelines for Exercise Testing and Prescription* (6th Ed.). Baltimore: Williams & Wilkins, 2000, pp. 322–351.

11. Franklin, B.A., K. Bonzheim, S. Gordon, and G.C. Timmis. Safety of medically supervised outpatient cardiac rehabilitation exercise therapy: a 16 year follow-up. *Chest* 114:902–906, 1998.

12. Franklin, B.A., J.M. Conviser, B. Stewart, J. Lasch, and G.C. Timmis. Sporadic exercise: a trigger for acute cardiovascular events? (Abstract). *Circulation* 102(Suppl. 2):II612, 2000.

13. Groeneveld, P.W., J.L. Kwong, Y. Liu, et al. Cost-effectiveness of automated external defibrillators on airlines. *JAMA* 286:1482–1489, 2001.

14. Haskell, W.L. Cardiovascular complications during exercise training of cardiac patients. *Circulation* 57:920–924, 1978.

15. Hossack, K.F., and R. Hartwig. Cardiac arrest associated with supervised cardiac rehabilitation. *J. Cardiac Rehabil.* 2:402–408, 1982.

16. International Health, Racquet, and Sportsclub Association. 2000 Profiles in Success. Boston, 1999.

17. Marenco, J.P., P.J. Wang, M.S. Link, M.K. Homoud, and N.A.M. Estes. Improving survival from sudden cardiac arrest: the role of the automated external defibrillator. *JAMA* 285:1193–1200, 2001.

18. McInnis, K.J., W. Herbert, D. Herbert, J. Herbert, P. Ribisl, and B. Franklin. Low compliance with national standards for cardiovascular emergency preparedness at health clubs. *Chest* 120:283–288, 2000.

19. Page, R.L., J.A. Joglar, R.C. Kowal, et al. Use of automated external defibrillators by a U.S. airline. *N. Engl. J. Med.* 343: 1210–1216, 2000.

20. Valenzuela, T.D., D.J. Roe, G. Nichol, L.L. Clark, D.W. Spaite, and R.G. Hardman. Outcomes of rapid defibrillation by security officers after cardiac arrest in casinos. *N. Engl. J. Med.* 343:1206–1209, 2000.

21. Van Camp, S.P., and R.A. Peterson. Cardiovascular complications of outpatient cardiac rehabilitation programs. *JAMA* 256: 1160–1163, 1986.

22. Williams, M. (ed.). *American Association for Cardiovascular, and Pulmonary Rehabilitation: Guidelines for Cardiac Rehabilitation and Secondary Prevention Programs.* Champaign, IL: Human Kinetics, 1999.

ACSM/AHA Joint Position Statement

Exercise and Acute Cardiovascular Events: Placing the Risks into Perspective

This joint position paper was authored by the American College of Sports Medicine and the American Heart Association. The content appears in AHA style. This paper is being published concurrently in *Medicine & Science in Sports & Exercise* and in *Circulation*.

0195-9131/07/3905-0886/0

Medicine & Science in Sports & Exercise®

This pronouncement was written for the American College of Sports Medicine by Paul D. Thompson, MD, FAHA (co-chair); Barry A. Franklin, PhD, FAHA (co-chair); Gary J. Balady, MD, FAHA; Steven N. Blair, PED, FAHA; Domenico Corrado, MD, PhD; N.A. Mark Estes III, MD, FAHA; Janet E. Fulton, PhD; Neil F. Gordon, MD, PhD, MPH; William L. Haskell, PhD, FAHA; Mark S. Link, MD; Barry J. Maron, MD; Murray A. Mittleman, MD, FAHA; Antonio Pelliccia, MD; Nanette K. Wenger, MD, FAHA; Stefan N. Willich, MD, FAHA; and Fernando Costa, MD, FAHA.

ABSTRACT

Habitual physical activity reduces coronary heart disease events, but vigorous activity can also acutely and transiently increase the risk of sudden cardiac death and acute myocardial infarction in susceptible persons. This scientific statement discusses the potential cardiovascular complications of exercise, their pathological substrate, and their incidence and suggests strategies to reduce these complications. Exercise-associated acute cardiac events generally occur in individuals with structural cardiac disease. Hereditary or congenital cardiovascular abnormalities are predominantly responsible for cardiac events among young individuals, whereas atherosclerotic disease is primarily responsible for these events in adults. The absolute rate of exercise-related sudden cardiac death varies with the prevalence of disease in the study population. The incidence of both acute myocardial infarction and sudden death is greatest in the habitually least physically active individuals. No strategies have been adequately studied to evaluate their ability to reduce exercise-related acute cardiovascular events. Maintaining physical fitness through regular physical activity may help to reduce events because a disproportionate number of events occur in least physically active subjects performing unaccustomed physical activity. Other strategies, such as screening patients before participation in exercise, excluding high-risk patients from certain activities, promptly evaluating possible prodromal symptoms, training fitness personnel for emergencies, and encouraging patients to avoid high-risk activities, appear prudent but have not been systematically evaluated.

Regular physical activity is widely advocated by the medical community in part because substantial epidemiological, clinical, and basic science evidence suggests that physical activity and exercise training delay the development of atherosclerosis and reduce the incidence of coronary heart disease (CHD) events (1–4). Nevertheless, vigorous physical activity can also acutely and transiently increase the risk of acute myocardial infarction (AMI) and sudden cardiac death (SCD) in susceptible individuals (5–7). This scientific statement presents the cardiovascular complications of vigorous exercise, their pathophysiological substrate, and their incidence in specific patient groups and evaluates strategies directed at reducing these complications. The goal is to provide healthcare professionals with the information they need to advise patients more accurately about the benefits and risks of physical activity.

Most studies of exercise-related cardiovascular events have examined events associated with sports participation in young subjects and with vigorous exercise in adults. Vigorous exercise is usually defined as an absolute exercise work rate of at least 6 metabolic equivalents (METs), which is historically assumed to equal an oxygen uptake ($\dot{V}O_2$) of 21 mL·kg^{-1}·min^{-1}. Six METs approximates the energy requirements of activities such as jogging. Six METs is an arbitrary threshold and does not account for the fact that the myocardial oxygen demands of any physical activity are more closely related to the $\dot{V}O_2$ requirements relative to maximal exercise capacity than to the absolute work rate per se. Consequently, exercise work rates < 6 METs may still place considerable stress on the cardiovascular systems of unfit and older individuals.

PATHOPHYSIOLOGICAL BASIS FOR EXERTION-RELATED CARDIOVASCULAR EVENTS

Exercise-associated acute cardiac events generally occur in individuals with structural cardiac disease.

Pathological Findings in Young Individuals

Among young individuals, variously defined as < 30 or < 40 years of age, the most frequent pathological findings are hereditary or congenital cardiovascular abnormalities (8–10), including hypertrophic cardiomyopathy; coronary artery anomalies (e.g., anomalous coronary artery origin, acute angle takeoff and ostial ridges, or intramyocardial course) (11,12); aortic stenosis; aortic dissection and rupture

probably associated with connective tissue defects such as Marfan syndrome; mitral valve prolapse; arrhythmogenic right ventricular cardiomyopathy; and arrhythmias, including those resulting from accessory atrioventricular pathways and channelopathies such as the long-QT syndrome. Myocarditis also is associated with exercise-related deaths in young individuals. Ventricular arrhythmias are the immediate cause of death in these conditions, except for Marfan syndrome, in which aortic rupture is often the proximate cause (Table 1).

Pathological Findings in Adults

In contrast to young subjects, coronary artery disease (CAD) is the most frequent pathological finding among older individuals who die during exertion (13,14). Among previously asymptomatic adults, evidence of acute coronary artery plaque disruption, including plaque rupture or erosion, with acute thrombotic occlusion is common (14). The mechanism by which vigorous exercise provokes such events is not defined, but suggested triggering mechanisms (15,16) include increased wall stress from increases in heart rate and blood pressure, exercise-induced coronary artery spasm in diseased artery segments (17), and increased flexing of atherosclerotic epicardial coronary arteries (15), leading to plaque disruption and thrombotic occlusion. Vigorous exercise also could provoke acute coronary thrombosis by deepening existing coronary fissures, augmenting catecholamine-induced platelet aggregation, or both. Spontaneous coronary plaque fissures are common and have been reported in 9% of subjects dying in motor vehicle accidents or by suicide and in 17% of people dying of noncoronary atherosclerosis (18). This observation suggests that mildly fissured coronary plaques require some exacerbating event such as vigorous physical activity to induce coronary thrombosis. An increase in thrombogenicity also could contribute to coronary thrombosis after plaque rupture or erosion. Increased platelet activation has been reported in sedentary individuals who engage in unaccustomed high-intensity exercise but not in physically conditioned individuals (19,20). Because circulating catecholamine levels are related more closely to the relative intensity of exercise for the individual than to the absolute exercise intensity, it is likely that platelet activation also is related to the relative intensity of the exercise session (21).

Among individuals with symptomatic CHD, pathophysiological processes may include plaque disruption as above or ischemia-induced ventricular fibrillation from peri-infarction, ischemic tissue,

TABLE 1 Cardiovascular Causes of Exercise-Related SCD in Young Athletes*

	Van Camp et al. (8) (n = 100),† %	Maron et al. (9) (n = 134), %	Corrado et al. (25) (n = 55),‡ %
Hypertrophic cardiomyopathy	51	36	1
Probable hypertrophic cardiomyopathy	5	10	
Coronary anomalies§	18	23	9
Valvular and subvalvular aortic stenosis	8	4	
Possible myocarditis	7	3	5
Dilated and nonspecific cardiomyopathy	7	3	1
Atherosclerotic CAD	3	2	10
Aortic dissection/rupture	2	5	1
Arrhythmogenic right ventricular cardiomyopathy	1	3	11
Myocardial scarring		3	
Mitral valve prolapse	1	2	6
Other congenital abnormalities		1.5	
Long-QT syndrome		0.5	1
Wolff-Parkinson-White syndrome	1		1
Cardiac conduction disease			3
Cardiac sarcoidosis		0.5	
Coronary artery aneurysm	1		
Normal heart at necropsy	7	2	1
Pulmonary thromboembolism			1

* Ages ranged from 13 to 24 (8), 12 to 40 (9), and 12 to 35 years (25) for the 3 studies, respectively. Van Kamp et al. (8) and Maron et al. (9) used the same database and include many of the same athletes. All (8), 90% (9), and 89% (25) had symptom onset during or within 1 hour of training or competition.
† Total exceeds 100% because several athletes had multiple abnormalities.
‡ Includes some athletes whose deaths were not associated with recent exertion.
§ Includes aberrant artery origin and course, tunneled arteries, and other abnormalities.

or scar (22). Vigorous physical exertion, which increases myocardial oxygen demand and simultaneously shortens diastole and coronary perfusion time, may induce myocardial ischemia and malignant cardiac arrhythmias. Reduced coronary perfusion can be exacerbated by a decrease in venous return secondary to abrupt cessation of activity, which possibly explains the clinical observation that collapse not infrequently occurs immediately after exercise. Ischemia can alter depolarization, repolarization, and conduction velocity and thereby trigger threatening ventricular arrhythmias (Fig. 1). In addition, myocardial ischemia (23), sodium-potassium shifts with exercise, increased catecholamine levels, and circulating free fatty acids may all increase the risks of ventricular arrhythmias (24).

THE IMPORTANCE OF AGE AND PATHOLOGICAL SUBSTRATE

The present scientific statement addresses the risks of exercise in both young and adult individuals, but it is critically important to recognize that these age groups have markedly different causes of exercise-related deaths and therefore markedly different

risk-to-benefit ratios for vigorous exercise. The causes of exercise-related events are not strictly separated by age, given that, for example, some young individuals with genetic defects in the low-density lipoprotein receptor may develop premature CAD, whereas some older individuals may present with structural congenital cardiac abnormalities. Nevertheless, the predominant pathological cause of exercise-related events in adults is occult CAD. Habitual vigorous physical activity appears to reduce the incidence of CHD events, and cardiac rehabilitation appears to reduce the risk of CHD death in patients with diagnosed disease, although neither conclusion has been proved by a randomized, controlled clinical trial. Thus, the benefits of physical activity in those with or at risk for CHD appear to outweigh the risks.

This situation is markedly different in young individuals with diagnosed or occult heart disease. Such subjects rarely die of CHD during exercise, and the clinical course of the responsible conditions such as hypertrophic cardiomyopathy and anomalous coronary arteries is not improved by vigorous exercise. Consequently, in populations with these diagnosed or occult cardiac diseases, the health risks of vigorous physical activity almost certainly

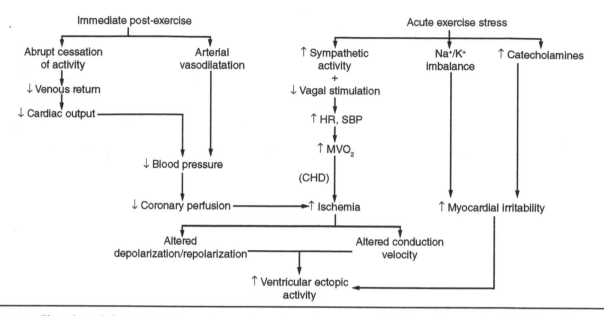

Figure 1 Physiological alterations accompanying acute exercise and recovery and their possible sequelae. HR indicates heart rate; SBP, systolic blood pressure; and MVO_2, myocardial oxygen uptake.

Reprinted, by permission, from B.A. Franklin, 1983, "The role of electrocardiographic monitoring in cardiac exercise programs," *Journal of Cardiopulmonary Rehabilitation* 3: 806-810.

exceed the benefits. Moderate physical activity may be justified in such patients on the basis of social and self-image considerations, as well as the benefits of physical activity in preventing obesity, obesity-related health problems, and atherosclerosis, all of which would further exacerbate the individual's cardiac risk.

INCIDENCE OF EXERCISE-RELATED ACUTE CARDIOVASCULAR EVENTS

The absolute risk of an exercise-related cardiovascular event varies with the prevalence of diagnosed or occult cardiac disease in the study population but appears to be extremely low in ostensibly healthy subjects. Because of the rarity of exercise-related cardiovascular events, studies examining its incidence are limited by small sample sizes and large confidence intervals. In addition, small changes in the number of events can produce large changes in the calculated incidence. Given these caveats, estimates are available for various patient groups.

Young Athletes

Van Camp and colleagues (8) estimated an absolute rate of exercise-related death among high school and college athletes of only 1 per 133,000 men and 1 per 769,000 women. These estimates include all sports-related non-traumatic deaths and are not restricted to cardiovascular events. A prospective, population-based study from Italy reported an incidence of ≈ 1 sudden death per 33,000 young athletes

per year (25). The rate may be higher because of the higher mean age (23 versus 16 years) of the Italian athletes, participation in sports with higher levels of exercise intensity in Italy, and the inclusion of all events, not just those directly associated with active physical exertion, in the Italian study.

Healthy Adults

Malinow and colleagues (26) reported only 1 acute cardiovascular event per 2,897,057 person-hours of physical activity among participants at YMCA sports centers. Vander and associates (27) reported only 1 nonfatal and 1 fatal event per 1 124,200 and 887,526 hours, respectively, of recreational physical activity. Gibbons and colleagues (28) reported only 1 nonfatal event during 187,399 hours of exercise, which corresponds to maximal risk estimates of 0.3 to 2.7 and 0.6 to 6.0 events per 10,000 person-hours for men and women, respectively. Thompson and collaborators (29) estimated only 1 death per 396,000 person-hours of jogging or 1 death per year for every 7620 joggers. Because half of the victims had known or readily diagnosed CHD, the estimated hourly and annual rates for previously healthy individuals were 1 death per 792,000 hours and 15,260 subjects, respectively. Siscovick and colleagues (5) estimated a similar annual rate of exercise-related cardiac arrest among previously healthy persons of 1 per 18,000 men. Both studies have wide confidence limits because the rates were calculated with only 10 (Thompson et al. (29)) and 9 (Siscovick et al. (5)) exercise-related deaths. All victims in both studies were men, and there are few estimates of event rates among women. The reasons for the rarity of exercise-related deaths among adult women are not clear but may relate to the delayed development of CHD in women and a lower rate of participation in vigorous exercise among older women. More recently, a database consisting of > 2.9 million members of a large commercial health/fitness facility chain reported 71 deaths (mean age, 52 ± 13 years; 61 men, 10 women) over a 2-year period, yielding 1 death per 82,000 members and a rate of 1 death per 2.57 million workouts (30). Nearly half of the exercise-related deaths were among members who exercised infrequently or less than once a week.

Vigorous exercise can also precipitate AMI (6,31,32), but even less precise estimates of the absolute incidence are available for this complication in the general population. Among 3617 men selected to participate in the Lipid Research Clinics Primary Prevention Trial because of hypercholesterolemia (plasma cholesterol ≥ 6.85 mmol/L [265 mg/dL] and low-density lipoprotein cholesterol ≥ 4.91 mmol/L [190 mg/dL]), 62 (1.7%) sustained an AMI (n = 54) or SCD (n = 8) definitely related to exertion during a mean follow-up of 7.4 years (33). An additional 225 men had acute events definitely not related to exercise, but the activity of another 170 men at the onset of their event was unclear. Nevertheless, these results suggest that the annual rate of exercise-related cardiovascular events among high-risk individuals may be substantial, with 0.2% of hypercholesterolemic men having an exercise-related event annually. The risk of exercise-related AMI also may be substantial in the general population. If we use the estimated incidence of SCD among healthy subjects from Rhode Island (29) and the observation that exercise-related AMI is 6.75 times more frequent than SCD (33), the annual incidence of exercise-related AMI could range from 1 AMI per 593 to 1 per 3852 apparently healthy middle-aged men.

Individuals with Diagnosed CHD

The incidence of exercise-related cardiovascular complications among persons with documented CHD has been estimated by at least 5 reports with data derived from exercise-based cardiac rehabilitation programs (34–38). Haskell (34) surveyed 30 cardiac rehabilitation programs in North America and reported 1 nonfatal and 1 fatal cardiovascular complication per 34,673 and 116,402 hours, respectively. The rate appears lower in contemporary exercise-based cardiac rehabilitation programs (Table 2) because an analysis of 4 reports estimates 1 cardiac arrest per 116,906 patient-hours, 1 myocardial infarction per 219,970 patient-hours, 1 fatality per 752,365 patient-hours, and 1 major complication per 81,670 patient-hours of participation (35–38). This low fatality rate applies only to medically supervised programs that are equipped to handle emergencies because the death rate would be 6-fold higher without the successful management of cardiac arrest (35–38). Furthermore, patients typically are medically evaluated before participation, which could decrease event rates, as could the serial surveillance provided by rehabilitation staff. Such considerations support the use of supervised exercise-based cardiac rehabilitation programs for patients after acute cardiac events.

DOES EXERCISE INCREASE THE RISK OF ACUTE CARDIOVASCULAR EVENTS?

Compelling evidence indicates that vigorous physical activity acutely increases the risk of cardiovascular events among young individuals and adults with both occult and diagnosed heart disease (5,7,25,29).

TABLE 2 Summary of Contemporary Exercise–Based Cardiac Rehabilitation Program Complication Rates

Investigator	Year	Patient-exercise hours	Cardiac arrest	MI	Fatal events	Major complications*
Van Camp and Peterson (35)	1980–1984	2,351,916	1/111,996†	1/293,990	1/783,972	1/81,101
Digenio et al. (36)	1982–1988	480,000	1/120,000‡	1/160,000	1/120,000	
Vongvanich et al. (38)	1986–1995	268,503	1/89,501§	1/268,503§	0/268,503	1/67,126
Franklin et al. (37)	1982–1998	292,254	1/146,127§	1/97,418§	0/292,254	1/58,451
Average			1/116,906	1/219,970	1/752,365	1/81,670

* MI and cardiac arrest.
† Fatal, 14%.
‡ Fatal, 75%.
§ Fatal, 0%.

Young Athletes

Corrado and colleagues (25) prospectively collected reports of SCDs among individuals 12 to 35 years of age over a 21-year period in the Veneto region of Italy. There were 2.3 and 0.9 SCDs per year per 100,000 athletes and nonathletes, respectively, or a 2.5-fold higher risk among the athletes (25). The death rate was higher among athletes despite the fact that all Italian athletes are required by law to undergo cardiovascular screening before participation (39). This report was not limited to SCD during exertion; therefore, the increased death rate among athletes cannot be attributed to exercise alone.

Healthy Adults

Studies in adults also suggest that exercise acutely increases the risk of cardiovascular events, despite a reduction in CHD with habitual physical activity. Both the Rhode Island study of exercise-related deaths (29) and the Seattle study of exercise-related cardiac arrests (5) report a higher estimated hourly death rate during exertion than during more leisurely activities. In Rhode Island, the SCD rate was 7.6 times the hourly death rate during sedentary activities (29). In Seattle, among previously asymptomatic individuals, the incidence of cardiac arrest during exercise was 25-fold higher than the incidence at rest or during lighter activity. The relative risk was greatest in the least compared with the most physically active men (56 and 5 times greater among the least and most active men, respectively) (5).

There is a similar pattern of increased risk with low levels of habitual activity for exercise-related AMI. Vigorous physical activity has been reported within 1 hour of AMI in 4% to 10% of AMI patients (6,31,32). This rate is 2.1 (Willich et al. (31)) to 10.1

(Giri et al. (6)) times higher than the rate during sedentary activities. As with SCD, the relative risk varies inversely with habitual physical activity and is greatest in the least physically active individuals. For patients with CHD, the relative risk of cardiac arrest during vigorous exercise is estimated as 6 to 164 times greater than expected without exertion (22).

Collectively, these data (Table 3) (5–7,29,31,32,40,41) suggest that vigorous exertion transiently increases the risk of AMI and SCD, particularly among habitually sedentary persons with occult or known CAD performing unaccustomed, vigorous physical activity. In fact, the Onset Study estimated that the risk of AMI during or soon after vigorous exertion was 50 times higher for the least active than for the most active cohort (Fig. 2) (32).

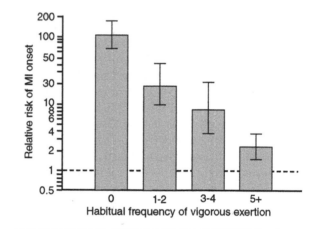

Figure 2 Relative risk of MI associated with vigorous exertion (≥ 6 METs) according to habitual frequency of vigorous exertion. The T bars indicate 95% confidence limits. The dotted line indicates risk of MI with no prior vigorous exertion.

Adapted, by permission, from M.A. Mittleman, 2005, "Triggering acute myocardial infarction by heavy physical exertion: Protection against triggering by regular exertion," *The New England Journal of Medicine* 329(23):1677-1683.

TABLE 3	Physical Stress as a Trigger of Acute Cardiovascular Events During Vigorous Exertion*		
Study	Effect period	End point	RR (95% CI)
Seattle study (5) (1984)	< 1 h	Primary cardiac arrest	56 (23–131)†
Onset study (32) (1993)	1 h	Nonfatal MI	5.9 (4.6–7.7)
TRIMM study (31) (1993)	1 h	Nonfatal MI	2.1 (1.1–3.6)
Hartford Hospital AMI study (6) (1999)	1 h	Nonfatal MI	10.1 (1.6–55.6)
SHEEP study (40) (2000)	< 15 min	Nonfatal MI	6.1 (4.2–9.0)
Physician's Health Study (7) (2000)	30 min	SCD	16.9 (10.5–27)

RR indicates relative risk and compares the risk of the cardiac event during exertion with that during sedentary activities; TRIMM, Triggers and Mechanisms of Myocardial Infarction Study; and SHEEP, Stockholm Heart Epidemiology Programme.

* Vigorous exertion is exercise intensity ≥ 6 METs (1 MET = 3.5 mL · kg⁻¹ · min⁻¹).

† This RR (56) is the exertion RR for habitually sedentary men. The RR (vs no prior vigorous exercise) for the most active men (≥ 140 min/wk vigorous exertion) was 5 (95% CI, 2 to 14).

Adapted, by permission, from M.A. Mittleman, 2005, "Trigger of acute cardiac events: New insights," *American Journal of Medicine In Sports* 4: 99-102.

RELATIVE RISK OF CARDIOVASCULAR EVENTS DURING EXERCISE VERSUS TOTAL RISK

Vigorous exercise increases the risk of a cardiovascular event during or soon after exertion in both young subjects with inherited cardiovascular disease and adults with occult or diagnosed CHD. Nevertheless, no evidence suggests that the risks of physical activity outweigh the benefits for healthy subjects. Indeed, the converse appears to be true. In the Seattle study, the relative risk of cardiac arrest was greater during exercise than at rest for all levels of habitual physical activity, but the total incidence of cardiac arrest, both at rest and during exercise, decreased with increasing exercise levels (5). Specifically, the overall incidence decreased from 18 events per 1 million person-hours in the least active to only 5 in the most active subjects. The risk of an exercise-related AMI also decreases with increasing amounts of physical activity (6,31,32). Considerable other epidemiological evidence, albeit no random-assignment, controlled study, supports the concept that regular physical activity, including vigorous activity, reduces CHD events over time (3).

In contrast to adults in whom vigorous exercise appears to reduce the overall risk of CHD, exercise in young subjects with occult cardiovascular disease may increase both exercise- and non-exercise-related sudden death. SCD during exertion in a young athlete results from the interaction between the underlying heart disease or substrate and the acute trigger of exertion plus other possible triggers associated with exercise, including emotional stress, hemodynamic changes, altered parasympathetic tone, and myocardial ischemia. Athletic training itself may increase the risk of sudden death in the young athlete with heart disease by altering the substrate. This alteration could occur by promoting disease progression or by increasing the risk of cardiac arrhythmia by structural or electrical changes. For example, in patients with hypertrophic cardiomyopathy, recurrent episodes of exercise-induced myocardial ischemia during intensive training could produce cell death and myocardial replacement fibrosis, which in turn enhance ventricular electrical instability. In patients with arrhythmogenic right ventricular cardiomyopathy, regular and intense physical activity could provoke right ventricular volume overload and cavity enlargement, which in turn may accelerate fibrofatty atrophy. In Marfan syndrome, the hemodynamic stress placed on the aorta by increased blood pressure and stroke volume during intense activity could increase the rate of aortic enlargement, thereby increasing the risk of aortic rupture. Consequently, the risk-to-benefit ratio of exercise differs between young and older subjects with occult cardiovascular disease.

The Risk of Special Situations and Activities

The rarity of exercise-related events makes the examination of special situations and activities difficult because of small sample sizes.

Morning Versus Afternoon Exercise

AMI and SCD in adults are more frequent in the early morning hours. This has prompted speculation as to whether vigorous exercise should be best restricted to afternoon hours in individuals at increased risk.

Young athletes. In contrast to adults, sudden death and cardiac arrest among young athletes occur primarily in the afternoon and early evening and are associated with training and competition (9). However, sudden death among nonathlete patients with hypertrophic cardiomyopathy is more frequent in the early waking hours, much like CHD (42). The explanation for this observation is not clear, and the timing of cardiac events in other young subjects with inherited cardiac disease is not known.

Adults. Murray and colleagues (43) found 5 cardiovascular events in 168,111 patient-hours of supervised cardiac rehabilitation exercise in the morning (3.0 events per 100,000 patient-hours) and 2 events during the 84,491 patient-hours of afternoon exercise (2.4 events per 100,000 patient-hours). This difference was not significant, but conclusions are limited by the number of subjects and available events. Similarly, Franklin and collaborators (37) reported that time of day had little or no influence on the rate of cardiovascular complications during exercise-based cardiac rehabilitation. Given the likely benefits of exercise in reducing cardiovascular events and the low overall rate of exercise-related events, it is probably more important that individuals exercise regularly at a convenient time of day than at a specific time of day.

High-Risk Activities

Few systematic studies have identified high-risk activities, again because of the rarity of exercise-related cardiovascular events. In general, the risk of any vigorous physical activity is an interaction of the exercise per se and the individual's physical fitness because identical physical tasks evoke lower cardiac demands in physically fit subjects than in unfit persons. Snow shoveling has repeatedly been associated with increased cardiovascular events (44,45), probably because it can elicit higher rate-pressure products than does treadmill exercise testing (46), because it is often performed out of necessity by unfit individuals, and because some cardiac patients develop angina at lower rate-pressure products, suggesting a coronary vasoconstrictor response, during exercise in cold temperatures (47).

STRATEGIES TO REDUCE EXERCISE-RELATED CARDIOVASCULAR EVENTS

No strategies have been adequately studied to evaluate their ability to reduce exercise-related acute cardiovascular events. Physicians should not overestimate the risks of exercise because the benefits of habitual physical activity substantially outweigh the risks. From observational studies (4), it appears that one of the most important defenses against exercise-related cardiovascular events in adults is to maintain physical fitness via regular physical activity because a disproportionate number of exercise events occur in the least physically active subjects performing unaccustomed vigorous physical activity (5,6,32). Several strategies to reduce events appear prudent although unproven. These include the following: preparticipation screening, excluding high-risk patients from some activities, reporting and evaluating prodromal symptoms, preparing fitness personnel and facilities for cardiovascular emergencies, and recommending prudent exercise programs. Each of these is discussed below.

Preparticipation Screening

Young athletes. The American Heart Association (AHA) recommends cardiovascular screening for high school and college athletes before athletic participation and at 2- to 4-year intervals (48,49). The examination should include a personal and family history and a physical examination focused on detecting conditions associated with exercise-related events (48). The AHA does not recommend routine, additional noninvasive testing such as a routine ECG. The omission of routine noninvasive testing is controversial because the Study Group on Sports Cardiology of the European Society of Cardiology has recommended that routine ECGs be obtained on all athletes as part of a preparticipation evaluation (50).

The European recommendation is based largely on an observational study performed in the Veneto region of Italy (51). Italy has mandated the prepar-

ticipation screening of athletes, including an ECG, since 1982. The annual incidence of sudden death among athletes 12 to 35 years of age decreased 89% with screening, from 3.6 deaths to 0.4 deaths per 100,000 athletes. There was no change in deaths among nonathletes, which suggests that screening mediated the decrease. These results provide the best evidence to date in support of the preparticipation screening of athletes but have several limitations (52). The study did not directly compare the screening and nonscreening of athletes but was a population-based, observational study. Other changes in the management of the athletes could have contributed to the improvement. In addition, the study did not directly compare screening performed with and without an ECG. Finally, there could be small differences in the screened and comparison populations because the athletes were screened at the Padua Center for Sports Medicine, whereas the comparison population consisted of subjects from the larger Veneto region.

Healthy adults. Although no data from controlled trials are available to guide the use of exercise testing in asymptomatic adults without known or suspected CAD before beginning an exercise training program, the writing groups from the American College of Cardiology (ACC)/AHA Guidelines on Exercise Testing (53) and the American College of Sports Medicine (ACSM) (54) have addressed this important issue by consensus. Although each group provides slightly different specific recommendations (see Table 4), the main theme of these recommendations is unified and clear: Individuals who appear to be at greater risk of having underlying CAD should be considered for exercise testing before beginning a vigorous ($\geq 60\%$ $\dot{V}O_2$ reserve) exercise training program (where $\dot{V}O_2$ reserve = percent intensity $\times$ [$\dot{V}O_2$ peak – $\dot{V}O_2$ rest] + $\dot{V}O_2$ rest). This is particularly evident in that both groups recommend exercise testing before exercise training for patients with diabetes mellitus. In contrast, the US Preventive Services Task Force (USPSTF) states that insufficient evidence exists to determine the benefits and harm of exercise stress testing before exercise programs (55).

A major limitation of exercise testing is that "positive" exercise test results require the presence of a flow-limiting coronary lesion, whereas most acute cardiac events in previously asymptomatic subjects are due to vulnerable plaque disruption. Consequently, an exercise stress test with or without imaging can be normal despite the presence of coronary plaque that may rupture. This requires that health professionals evaluate the entire ath-

TABLE 4	ACC/AHA, ACSM, and USPSTF Recommendations for Exercise Testing Before Exercise Training		
ACC/AHA	**ACSM**	**USPSTF**
Asymptomatic persons with diabetes mellitus who plan to start vigorous exercise (Class IIa)	Asymptomatic persons with diabetes mellitus (or other metabolic disease) who plan to start moderate (40% to 59% o2 reserve) to vigorous (≥ 60% o2 reserve) exercise	Recommends against routine exercise testing of low-risk adults in general and finds insufficient evidence for exercise testing before exercise training
Asymptomatic men > 45 y of age and women > 55 y of age who plan to start vigorous exercise (Class IIb)	Asymptomatic men > 45 y of age and women > 55 y of age or those who meet the threshold for > 2 risk factors who plan to start vigorous exercise	

ACC/AHA Class IIa indicates that the weight of evidence/opinion is in favor of usefulness/efficacy; Class IIb indicates that the usefulness/efficacy is less well established by evidence/opinion.
Reprinted, by permission, from R.J. Northcote, C. Flannigan, and D. Ballantyne, 1986, "Sudden death and vigorous exercise: A study of 60 deaths associated with squash," *British Heart Journal* 55: 198-203.

erosclerotic risk profile in patients when advising on the feasibility of a vigorous exercise program.

Exclusion of High-Risk Subjects

Cardiovascular screening necessitates a strategy of excluding high-risk subjects from athletic and vigorous exercise participation. Both the ACC/AHA (53) and the ACSM (54) recommend exercise testing before vigorous exercise training in persons with known cardiovascular disease.

Guidelines for determining eligibility for competitive athletics among children and adults have been presented in the 36th Bethesda Conference on this topic (56). These guidelines specifically address athletic competition but can be extrapolated to recommend or restrict vigorous exercise in patients with diagnosed cardiac conditions.

Reporting and Evaluating Possible Prodromal Symptoms

Several reports suggest that many individuals with exercise-related cardiovascular events had prodromal symptoms that were ignored by the victims or their physician. Of 134 young competitive athletes with SCD, 121 of whom (90%) died during or immediately after exertion, 24 (18%) experienced probable cardiac symptoms in the 36 months preceding death (9). Similarly, among adults, 50% of joggers (13), 75% of squash players (57), and 81% of distance runners (58) who died during exercise had probable cardiac symptoms before death (Table 5). Most reported these symptoms only to relatives, and few sought medical attention. Consequently, it is prudent for exercising adults to know the nature of prodromal cardiac symptoms and the need for prompt medical attention. In addition, physicians should carefully evaluate possible cardiac symptoms in physically active individuals. Both patients and physicians may ignore or not adequately evaluate symptoms in highly active

individuals in the mistaken belief that high levels of fitness protect against, rather than only reduce, the risk of cardiac disease.

Preparing Fitness Personnel and Exercise Facilities for Cardiovascular Emergencies

The death rate from exercise-related cardiovascular events might be reduced if personnel and facilities involved with exercise activities were prepared to handle cardiac emergencies. The AHA has recommended that coaches and trainers attending high school and college athletes be trained in cardiopulmonary resuscitation (48). The AHA and ACSM recommend that participants in fitness facilities be screened for heart disease with a specially designed questionnaire (59) and that facility staff be trained in managing cardiovascular emergencies. These organizations also have strongly encouraged fitness facilities to have automatic external defibrillators available for cardiac emergencies (60). The AHA and the ACSM have developed a preparticipation

TABLE 5	Prodromal Symptoms Reported by 45 Subjects Within 1 Week of Their SCD
Symptom	**Reports, n**
Chest pain/angina	15
Increasing fatigue	12
Indigestion/heartburn/gastrointestinal symptoms	10
Excessive breathlessness	6
Ear or neck pain	5
Vague malaise	5
Upper respiratory tract infection	4
Dizziness/palpitations	3
Severe headache	2

Reprinted, by permission, from R.J. Northcote, C. Flannigan, and D. Ballantyne, 1986, "Sudden death and vigorous exercise: A study of 60 deaths associated with squash," *British Heart Journal* 55: 198-203.

screening questionnaire for health-fitness facilities to identify individuals at risk from exercise (59). Nevertheless, a survey of 65 health clubs in Ohio revealed that 28% of the clubs failed to use pre-entry cardiac screenings, most had no written emergency response plans, > 90% failed to conduct emergency drills, and only 3% had an automatic external defibrillator (61). Although it is unclear whether these findings are typical of clubs nationwide, the results suggest that a significant gap exists between national recommendations and practices. At minimum, it would be prudent for health-fitness facilities to perform pre-entry screenings, to have written emergency policies, to conduct regular emergency drills and cardiopulmonary resuscitation practice, to have automatic external defibrillators available for immediate use by trained personnel (59), and to establish a "hotline" to summon emergency medical services.

RECOMMENDING PRUDENT EXERCISE PROGRAMS

Ostensibly healthy adults without known cardiac disease should be encouraged to develop gradually progressive exercise regimens. Because the least fit individuals are at greatest risk for exercise-related events, gradually progressive programs should theoretically increase fitness and reduce acute CAD events without excessive risk. Patients with known cardiac disease also should be counseled to include at least 5 minutes each of warm-up and cool-down in their exercise training sessions to reduce the likelihood of inducing cardiac ischemia with sudden, intense physical effort (62,63) and to avoid the decrease in central blood volume that can occur with the abrupt cessation of physical activity. Patients with cardiovascular disease who are interested in participating in competitive sports should be evaluated and advised in accordance with the 36th Bethesda Conference guidelines (56). Physically inactive individuals and patients with known cardiovascular disease should avoid strenuous, unaccustomed exercise in both excessively cold and hot environmental conditions. Vigorous exercise in the cold such as snow shoveling has repeatedly been associated with acute cardiovascular events (44,45,64), and hot, humid environments require an increased heart rate response to handle the increased thermal load (65). Increased altitude reduces oxygen availability and augments the cardiorespiratory and hemodynamic responses to a given submaximal work rate, thereby increasing cardiac demands. Individuals exercising at altitudes of > 1500 m should limit the intensity of their exercise until acclimatized (54,66).

SUMMARY

No sufficiently powered, randomized controlled studies have evaluated the contribution of exercise training to reducing CAD events. Nevertheless, a variety of epidemiological, basic scientific, and clinical evidence suggests that habitual physical activity decreases the risk of fatal and nonfatal CAD events and that the benefits of regular physical activity outweigh its risks. Consequently, physical activity should be encouraged for most individuals in accordance with the Centers for Disease Control and Prevention/ACSM recommendations for ≥ 30 minutes of moderate-intensity physical activity such as brisk walking on most, preferably all, days of the week (67,68). Vigorous exercise, however, transiently increases the risk of AMI and SCD, even in exercise-conditioned individuals, and several strategies are recommended to potentially reduce this risk:

- Healthcare professionals should know the pathological conditions associated with exercise-related events so that physically active children and adults can be appropriately evaluated.
- Active individuals should know the nature of cardiac prodromal symptoms and seek prompt medical care if such symptoms develop.
- High school and college athletes should undergo pre-participation screening by qualified professionals (49,69).
- Athletes with known cardiac conditions should be evaluated for competition according to published guidelines (56).
- Healthcare facilities should ensure that their staffs are trained in managing cardiac emergencies, have a specified plan, and have appropriate resuscitation equipment.
- Active individuals should modify their exercise programs in response to variations in their exercise capacity, their habitual activity level, and the environment.

Although these interventions have not been rigorously evaluated and documented to reduce exercise-related cardiovascular events, they appear prudent given our present understanding of the risks and benefits of exercise.

WRITING GROUP DISCLOSURES

Writing group member	Employment	Research grant	Other research support	Speakers' bureau/ honoraria	Ownership interest	Consultant/ advisory board	Other
Paul D. Thompson	Hartford Hospital	Merck; Pfizer; AstraZeneca; Kos Pharma	NIH Donaghue Foundation	Merck; Pfizer; Kos; Abbott; Reliant	AstraZeneca	AstraZeneca	None
Barry A. Franklin	William Beaumont Hospital	None	None	None	None	None	None
Gary J. Balady	Boston Medical Center	None	None	None	None	None	None
Steven N. Blair	Cooper Institute	None	None	None	None	None	None
Domenico Corrado	University of Padova	None	None	None	None	None	None
N.A. Mark Estes III	Tufts-New England Medical Center	None	None	Guidant*; Medtronic*; St Jude Medical*	None	Guidant*	None
Janet E. Fulton	Centers for Disease Control and Prevention	None	None	None	None	None	None
Neil F. Gordon	St Joseph's/ Candler Health System	None	None	None	INTERVENT USA, Inc†	None	None
William L. Haskell	Stanford Medical School	None	None	None	None	None	None
Mark S. Link	New England Medical Center	None	None	None	None	None	None
Barry J. Maron	Minneapolis Heart Institute Foundation	Medtronic	None	None	None	None	Minneapolis Heart Institute Foundation
Murray A. Mittleman	Beth Israel Deaconess Medical Center	None	None	None	None	None	None
Antonio Pelliccia	Institute of Sports Science	None	None	None	None	None	None
Nanette K. Wenger	Emory University	Eli Lilly†; AstraZeneca*	Pfizer Steering Committee†	Pfizer*; Novartis*; Merck*; Bristol-Myers Squibb*; Eli Lilly*	None	None	None
Stefan N. Willich	Humboldt University, Berlin	None	None	None	None	None	None
Fernando Costa‡	Reliant Pharmaceuticals	None	None	None	None		None

This table represents the relationships of writing group members that may be perceived as actual or reasonably perceived conflicts of interest as reported on the Disclosure Questionnaire, which all members of the writing group are required to complete and submit. A relationship is considered to be "significant" if (1) the person receives $10,000 or more during any 12-month period or 5% or more of the person's gross income or (2) the person owns 5% or more of the voting stock or share of the entity or owns $10,000 or more of the fair market value of the entity. A relationship is considered to be "modest" if it is less than "significant" under the preceding definition.

* Modest.   † Significant.   ‡ Dr Costa was affiliated with the American Heart Association at the time this statement was written.

REVIEWER DISCLOSURES

Reviewer	Employment	Research grant	Other research support	Speakers' bureau/ honoraria	Ownership interest	Consultant/ advisory board	Other
Elliott M. Antman	Brigham and Women's Hospital	None	None	None	None	None	None
Gerald Fletcher	Mayo Clinic Jacksonville	None	None	None	None	None	None
Carl Foster	University of Wisconsin- La Crosse	None	None	None	None	None	None
Benjamin D. Levine	University of Texas Southwestern Medical Center at Dallas	None	None	None	None	None	None

This table represents the relationships of reviewers that may be perceived as actual or reasonably perceived conflicts of interest as reported on the Disclosure Questionnaire, which all reviewers are required to complete and submit.

The American Heart Association makes every effort to avoid any actual or potential conflicts of interest that may arise as a result of an outside relationship or a personal, professional, or business interest of a member of the writing panel. Specifically, all members of the writing group are required to complete and submit a Disclosure Questionnaire showing all such relationships that might be perceived as real or potential conflicts of interest.

REFERENCES

1. Powell, K. E., P. D. Thompson, C. J. Caspersen, and J. S. Kendrick. Physical activity and the incidence of coronary heart disease. *Annu. Rev. Public Health* 8:253–287, 1987.

2. Fletcher, G. F., G. Balady, S. N. Blair, J. Blumenthal, C. Caspersen, B. Chaitman, S. Epstein, E. S. Sivarajan Froelicher, V. F. Froelicher, I. L. Pina, and M. L. Pollock. Statement on exercise: benefits and recommendations for physical activity programs for all Americans: a statement for health professionals by the Committee on Exercise and Cardiac Rehabilitation of the Council on Clinical Cardiology, American Heart Association. *Circulation* 94:857–862, 1996.

3. Lee, I. M., and R. S. Paffenbarger Jr. The role of physical activity in the prevention of coronary artery disease. In: *Exercise and Sports Cardiology*, P. D. Thompson. New York, NY: McGraw-Hill, 2001.

4. Thompson, P. D., D. Buchner, I. L. Pina, G. J. Balady, M. A. Williams, B. H. Marcus, K. Berra, S. N. Blair, F. Costa, B. Franklin, G. F. Fletcher, N. F. Gordon, R. R. Pate, B. L. Rodriguez, A. K. Yancey, N. K. Wenger, for the American Heart Association Council on Clinical Cardiology Subcommittee on Exercise, Rehabilitation, and Prevention; American Heart Association Council on Nutrition, Physical Activity, and Metabolism Subcommittee on Physical Activity. Exercise and physical activity in the prevention and treatment of atherosclerotic cardiovascular disease: a statement from the Council on Clinical Cardiology (Subcommittee on Exercise, Rehabilitation, and Prevention) and the Council on Nutrition, Physical Activity, and Metabolism (Subcommittee on Physical Activity). *Circulation* 107:3109–3116, 2003.

5. Siscovick, D. S., N. S. Weiss, R. H. Fletcher, and T. Lasky. The incidence of primary cardiac arrest during vigorous exercise. *N. Engl. J. Med.* 311:874–877, 1984.

6. Giri, S., P. D. Thompson, F. J. Kiernan, J. Clive, D. B. Fram, J. F. Mitchel, J. A. Hirst, R. G. McKay, and D. D. Waters. Clinical and angiographic characteristics of exertion-related acute myocardial infarction. *JAMA* 282:1731–1736, 1999.

7. Albert, C. M., M. A. Mittleman, C. U. Chae, I. M. Lee, C.H. Hennekens, and J. E. Manson. Triggering of sudden death from cardiac causes by vigorous exertion. *N. Engl. J. Med.* 343: 1355–1361, 2000.

8. Van Camp, S. P., C. M. Bloor, F. O. Mueller, R. C. Cantu, and H. G. Olson. Nontraumatic sports death in high school and college athletes. *Med. Sci. Sports Exerc.* 27:641–647, 1995.

9. Maron, B. J., J. Shirani, L. C. Poliac, R. Mathenge, W. C. Roberts, and F. O. Mueller. Sudden death in young competitive athletes: clinical, demographic, and pathological profiles. *JAMA* 276:199–204, 1996.

10. Corrado, D., G. Thiene, A. Nava, L. Rossi, and N. Pennelli. Sudden death in young competitive athletes: clinicopathologic correlations in 22 cases. *Am. J. Med.* 89:588–596, 1990.

11. Iskandar, E. G., and P. D. Thompson. Exercise-related sudden death due to an unusual coronary artery anomaly. *Med. Sci. Sports Exerc.* 36:180–182, 2004.

12. Virmani, R., P. K. Chun, R. E. Goldstein, M. Robinowitz, and H. A. McAllister. Acute takeoffs of the coronary arteries along the aortic wall and congenital coronary ostial valve-like ridges: association with sudden death. *J. Am. Coll. Cardiol.* 3:766–771, 1984.

13. Thompson, P. D., M. P. Stern, P. Williams, K. Duncan, W. L. Haskell, and P. D. Wood. Death during jogging or running: a study of 18 cases. *JAMA* 242:1265–1267, 1979.

14. Burke, A. P., A. Farb, G. T. Malcom, Y. Liang, J. E. Smialek, and R. Virmani. Plaque rupture and sudden death related to exertion in men with coronary artery disease. *JAMA* 281: 921–926, 1999.

15. Black, A., M. M. Black, and G. Gensini. Exertion and acute coronary artery injury. *Angiology* 26:759–783, 1975.

16. Thompson, P. D. The cardiovascular risks of exercise. In: *Exercise and Sports Cardiology*, P. D. Thompson. New York, NY: McGraw-Hill, 2001.

17. Gordon, J. B., P. Ganz, E. G. Nabel, R. D. Fish, J. Zebede, G. H. Mudge, R. W. Alexander, and A. P. Selwyn. Atherosclerosis influences the vasomotor response of epicardial coronary arteries to exercise. *J. Clin. Invest.* 83:1946–1952, 1989.

18. Davies, M. J., J. M. Bland, J. R. Hangartner, A. Angelini, and A. C. Thomas. Factors influencing the presence or absence of acute coronary artery thrombi in sudden ischaemic death. *Eur. Heart J.* 10:203–208, 1989.

19. Kestin, A. S., P. A. Ellis, M. R. Barnard, A. Errichetti, B. A. Rosner, and A. D. Michelson. Effect of strenuous exercise on platelet activation state and reactivity. *Circulation* 88(pt 1): 1502–1511, 1993.

20. Li, N., N. H. Wallen, and P. Hjemdahl. Evidence for prothrombotic effects of exercise and limited protection by aspirin. *Circulation* 100:1374–1379, 1999.

21. Rowell, L.B. *Human Circulation: Regulation During Physical Stress*, New York, NY: Oxford University Press, 1986.

22. Cobb, L. A., and W. D. Weaver. Exercise: a risk for sudden death in patients with coronary heart disease. *J. Am. Coll. Cardiol.* 7:215–219, 1986.

23. Hoberg, E., G. Schuler, B. Kunze, A. L. Obermoser, K. Hauer, H. P. Mautner, G. Schlierf, and W. Kubler. Silent myocardial ischemia as a potential link between lack of premonitoring symptoms and increased risk of cardiac arrest during physical stress. *Am. J. Cardiol.* 65:583–589, 1990.

24. Sejersted, O. M., and G. Sjogaard. Dynamics and consequences of potassium shifts in skeletal muscle and heart during exercise. *Physiol. Rev.* 80:1411–1481, 2000.

25. Corrado, D., C. Basso, G. Rizzoli, M. Schiavon, and G. Thiene. Does sports activity enhance the risk of sudden

death in adolescents and young adults? *J. Am. Coll. Cardiol.* 42:1959–1963, 2003.

26. Malinow, M., D. McGarry, and K. Kuehl. Is exercise testing indicated for asymptomatic active people? *J. Cardiac. Rehabilitation* 4:376–379, 1984.

27. Vander, L., B. Franklin, and M. Rubenfire. Cardiovascular complications of recreational physical activity. *Phys. Sportsmed.* 10:89–90, 1982.

28. Gibbons, L. W., K. H. Cooper, B. M. Meyer, and R. C. Ellison. The acute cardiac risk of strenuous exercise. *JAMA* 244: 1799–1801, 1980.

29. Thompson, P. D., E. J. Funk, R. A. Carleton, and W. Q. Sturner. Incidence of death during jogging in Rhode Island from 1975 through 1980. *JAMA* 247:2535–2538, 1982.

30. Franklin, B. A., J. M. Conviser, B. Stewart, J. Lasch, and G. C. Timmis. Sporadic exercise: a trigger for acute cardiovascular events? *Circulation* 102:II-612, 2005. Abstract.

31. Willich, S. N., M. Lewis, H. Lowel, H. R. Arntz, F. Schubert, and R. Schroder. Physical exertion as a trigger of acute myocardial infarction: Triggers and Mechanisms of Myocardial Infarction Study Group. *N. Engl. J. Med.* 329:1684–1690, 1993.

32. Mittleman, M. A., M. Maclure, G. H. Tofler, J. B. Sherwood, R. J. Goldberg, and J. E. Muller. Triggering of acute myocardial infarction by heavy physical exertion: protection against triggering by regular exertion. Determinants of Myocardial Infarction Onset Study Investigators. *N. Engl. J. Med.* 329:1677–1683, 1993.

33. Siscovick, D. S., L. G. Ekelund, J. L. Johnson, Y. Truong, and A. Adler. Sensitivity of exercise electrocardiography for acute cardiac events during moderate and strenuous physical activity: the Lipid Research Clinics Coronary Primary Prevention Trial. *Arch. Intern. Med.* 151:325–330, 1991.

34. Haskell, W. L. Cardiovascular complications during exercise training of cardiac patients. *Circulation* 57:920–924, 1978.

35. Van Camp, S. P., and R. A. Peterson. Cardiovascular complications of outpatient cardiac rehabilitation programs. *JAMA* 256:1160–1163, 1986.

36. Digenio, A. G., J. G. Sim, R. J. Dowdeswell, and R. Morris. Exercise-related cardiac arrest in cardiac rehabilitation: the Johannesburg experience. *S. Afr. Med. J.* 79:188–191, 1991.

37. Franklin, B. A., K. Bonzheim, S. Gordon, and G. C. Timmis. Safety of medically supervised outpatient cardiac rehabilitation exercise therapy: a 16-year follow-up. *Chest* 114:902–906, 1998.

38. Vongvanich, P., M. J. Paul-Labrador, and C. N. Merz. Safety of medically supervised exercise in a cardiac rehabilitation center. *Am. J. Cardiol.* 77:1383–1385, 1996.

39. Pelliccia, A., and B. J. Maron. Preparticipation cardiovascular evaluation of the competitive athlete: perspectives from the 30-year Italian experience. *Am. J. Cardiol.* 75:827–829, 1995.

40. Hallqvist, J., J. Moller, A. Ahlbom, F. Diderichsen, C. Reuterwall, and U. De Faire. Does heavy physical exertion trigger myocardial infarction? A case-crossover analysis nested in a population-based case-referent study. *Am. J. Epidemiol.* 151:459–467, 2000.

41. Mittleman, M. A. Trigger of acute cardiac events: new insights. *Am. J. Med. Sports* 4:99–102, 2005.

42. Maron, B. J., J. Kogan, M. A. Proschan, G. M. Hecht, and W. C. Roberts. Circadian variability in the occurrence of sudden cardiac death in patients with hypertrophic cardiomyopathy. *J. Am. Coll. Cardiol.* 23:1405–1409, 1994.

43. Murray, P. M., D. M. Herrington, C. W. Pettus, H. S. Miller, J. D. Cantwell, and W. C. Little. Should patients with heart disease exercise in the morning or afternoon? *Arch. Intern. Med.* 153:833–836, 1993.

44. Faich, G., and R. Rose. Blizzard morbidity and mortality: Rhode Island, 1978. *Am. J. Public Health* 69:1050–1052, 1979.

45. Hammoudeh, A. J., and J. I. Haft. Coronary-plaque rupture in acute coronary syndromes triggered by snow shoveling. *N. Engl. J. Med.* 335:2001, 1996.

46. Franklin, B. A., P. Hogan, K. Bonzheim, D. Bakalyar, E. Terrien, S. Gordon, and G. C. Timmis. Cardiac demands of heavy snow shoveling. *JAMA* 273:880–882, 1995.

47. Juneau, M., M. Johnstone, E. Dempsey, and D. D. Waters. Exercise-induced myocardial ischemia in a cold environment: effect of antianginal medications. *Circulation* 79:1015–1020, 1989.

48. Maron, B. J., P. D. Thompson, J. C. Puffer, C. A. McGrew, W. B. Strong, P. S. Douglas, L. T. Clark, M. J. Mitten, M. H. Crawford, D. L. Atkins, D. J. Driscoll, and A. E. Epstein. Cardiovascular preparticipation screening of competitive athletes: a statement for health professionals from the Sudden Death Committee (Clinical Cardiology) and Congenital Cardiac Defects Committee (Cardiovascular Disease in the Young), American Heart Association. *Circulation* 94:850–856, 1996.

49. Maron, B. J., P. D. Thompson, J. C. Puffer, C. A. McGrew, W. B. Strong, P. S. Douglas, L. T. Clark, M. J. Mitten, M. D. Crawford, D.L. Atkins, D. J. Driscoll, and A. E. Epstein. Cardiovascular preparticipation screening of competitive athletes: addendum: an addendum to a statement for health professionals from the Sudden Death Committee (Council on Clinical Cardiology) and the Congenital Cardiac Defects Committee (Council on Cardiovascular Disease in the Young), American Heart Association. *Circulation* 97:2294, 1998.

50. Corrado, D., A. Pelliccia, H. H. Bjornstad, L. Vanhees, A. Biffi, M. Borjesson, N. Panhuyzen-Goedkoop, A. Deligiannis, E. Solberg, D. Dugmore, K. P. Mellwig, D. Assanelli, P. Delise, F. Van Buuren, A. Anastasakis, H. Heidbuchel, E. Hoffmann, R. Fagard, S. G. Priori, C. Basso, E. Arbustini, C. Blomstromlundqvist, W. J. McKenna, G. Thiene, for the Study Group of Sport Cardiology of the Working Group of Cardiac Rehabilitation and Exercise Physiology and the Working Group of Myocardial and Pericardial Diseases of the European Society of Cardiology. Cardiovascular pre-participation screening of young competitive athletes for prevention of sudden death: proposal for a common European protocol: consensus statement of the Study Group of Sport Cardiology of the Working Group of Cardiac Rehabilitation and Exercise Physiology and the Working Group of Myocardial and Pericardial Diseases of the European Society of Cardiology. *Eur. Heart J.* 26:516–524, 2005.

51. Corrado, D., C. Basso, A. Pavei, P. Michieli, M. Schiavon, and G. Thiene. Trends in sudden cardiovascular death

in young competitive athletes after implementation of a preparticipation screening program. *JAMA* 296:1593–1601, 2006.

52. Thompson, P. D., and B. D. Levine. Protecting athletes from sudden cardiac death. *JAMA* 296:1648–1650, 2006.

53. Gibbons R. J., G. J. Balady, J. T. Bricker, B. R. Chaitman, G.F. Fletcher, V. F. Froelicher, D. B. Mark, B. D. McCallister, A. N. Mooss, M. G. O'Reilly, W. L. Winters Jr, E. M. Antman, J. S. Alpert, D. P. Faxon, V. Fuster, G. Gregoratos, L. F. Hiratzka, A. K. Jacobs, R. O. Russell, S. C. Smith Jr. ACC/AHA 2002 guideline update for exercise testing: a report of the American College of Cardiology/American Heart Association Task Force on Practice Guidelines (Committee on Exercise Testing). Available at: http://www.acc.org/clinical/guidelines/exercise/dirIndex.htm. Accessed May 23, 2005.

54. American College of Sports Medicine. *Guidelines for Exercise Testing and Prescription,* 7th ed, Baltimore, MD: Lippincott Williams & Wilkins, 2005.

55. US Preventive Services Task Force. Screening for coronary heart disease: recommendation statement. *Ann. Intern. Med.* 140:569–572, 2004.

56. Maron, B. J., and D. P. Zipes. 36th Bethesda Conference: eligibility recommendations for competitive athletes with cardiovascular abnormalities. *J. Am. Coll. Cardiol.* 45:2–64, 2005.

57. Northcote, R. J., C. Flannigan, and D. Ballantyne. Sudden death and vigorous exercise: a study of 60 deaths associated with squash. *Br. Heart J.* 55:198–203, 1986.

58. Noakes, T. D., L. H. Opie, and A. G. Rose. Marathon running and immunity to coronary heart disease: fact versus fiction. In: *Symposium on Cardiac Rehabilitation,* B. A. Franklin and M. Rubenfire. Philadelphia, PA: WB Saunders, 1984.

59. Balady, G. J., B. Chaitman, D. Driscoll, C. Foster, E. Froelicher, N. Gordon, R. Pate, J. Rippe, and T. Bazzarre. Recommendations for cardiovascular screening, staffing, and emergency policies at health/fitness facilities. *Circulation* 97:2283–2293, 1998.

60. Balady, G. J., B. Chaitman, C. Foster, E. Froelicher, N. Gordon, S. Van Camp, for the American Heart Association and American College of Sports Medicine. Automated external defibrillators in health/fitness facilities: supplement to the AHA/ACSM Recommendations for Cardiovascular Screening, Staffing, and Emergency Policies at Health/Fitness Facilities. *Circulation* 105:1147–1150, 2002.

61. McInnis, K., W. Herbert, D. Herbert, J. Herbert, P. Ribisl, and B. Franklin. Low compliance with national standards for cardiovascular emergency preparedness at health clubs. *Chest* 120:283–288, 2001.

62. Barnard, R. J., G. W. Gardner, N. V. Diaco, R. N. Macalpin, and A. A. Kattus. Cardiovascular responses to sudden strenuous exercise: heart rate, blood pressure, and ECG. *J. Appl. Physiol.* 34:833–837, 1973.

63. Barnard, R. J., R. Macalpin, A. A. Kattus, and G. D. Buckberg. Ischemic response to sudden strenuous exercise in healthy men. *Circulation* 48:936–942, 1973.

64. Glass, R. I., and M. M. Zack Jr. Increase in deaths from ischaemic heart-disease after blizzards. *Lancet* 1:485–487, 1979.

65. Pandolf, K. B., E. Cafarelli, B. J. Noble, and K. F. Metz. Hyperthermia: effect on exercise prescription. *Arch. Phys. Med. Rehabil.* 56:524–526, 1975.

66. Levine, B. D., J. H. Zuckerman, and C. R. DeFilippi. Effect of high-altitude exposure in the elderly: the Tenth Mountain Division study. *Circulation* 96:1224–1232, 1997.

67. Pate, R. R., M. Pratt, S. N. Blair, W. L. Haskell, C. A. Macera, C. Bouchard, D. Buchner, W. Ettinger, G. W. Heath, A. C. King, A. Kriska, A. S. Leon, B. H. Marcus, J. Morris, R. S. Paffenbarger, K. Patrick, M. L. Pollock, J.M. Rippe, J. Sallis, and J. H. Wilmore. Physical activity and public health: a recommendation from the Centers for Disease Control and Prevention and the American College of Sports Medicine. *JAMA* 273:402–407, 1995.

68. Mosca, L., L. J. Appel, E. J. Benjamin, K. Berra, N. Chandrastrobos, R. P. Fabunmi, D. Grady, C. K. Haan, S. N. Hayes, D. R. Judelson, N. L. Keenan, P. McBride, S. Oparil, P. Ouyang, M. C. Oz, M. E. Mendelsohn, R. C. Pasternak, V. W. Pinn, R. M. Robertson, K. Schenck-Gustafsson, C. A. Sila, S. C. Smith Jr, G. Sopko, A. L. Taylor, B. W. Walsh, N. K. Wenger, C. L. Williams, for the American Heart Association. Evidence-based guidelines for cardiovascular disease prevention in women. *Circulation* 109:672–693, 2004.

69. Maron, B. J., J. M. Gardin, J. M. Flack, S. S. Gidding, T.T. Kurosaki, and D. E. Bild. Prevalence of hypertrophic cardiomyopathy in a general population of young adults: echocardiographic analysis of 4111 subjects in the CARDIA Study: Coronary Artery Risk Development in (Young) Adults. *Circulation* 92:785–789, 1995.

70. Franklin, B. A. The role of electrocardiographic monitoring in cardiac exercise programs. *J. Cardiopulm. Rehabil.* 3:806–810, 1983.

Core Medical Fitness Association Standards for Medical Fitness Center Facilities

Medical Oversight

1. A medical fitness center must have medical oversight. A medical director, a physician advisory committee, and/or a physician advisor must be in place to provide medical oversight for the facility's programming in order to maximize the safety of all participants and ensure medically and scientifically sound programs and services.

2. The clinical programs and services offered within a medical fitness center must comply with the current requirements by the Centers for Medicare and Medicaid Services, such as cardiac rehabilitation phase II, physical and occupational therapy, speech therapy, and other billed clinical services, including, but not limited to, the requirements for physician referral, supervision, communication, documentation and charting, and patient safety.

3. A medical fitness center must demonstrate a direct and valid relationship with its community healthcare system and local continuum of care.

Pre-Activity Screening

1. A medical fitness center must offer each member an appropriate pre-activity screening process and refer moderate- to high-risk individuals to their respective physicians for medical clearance prior to participation.

2. If the pre-activity screening identifies a potential user as having a known cardiovascular, metabolic, or pulmonary disease and/or as a high-risk individual, the user should be advised, in writing, to consult with a physician and/or qualified healthcare provider and provide documentation of such consultation to the facility prior to participating in physical activity at the facility.

3. The pre-activity screening should be reviewed and interpreted by qualified staff and the results documented, including referral to a qualified healthcare provider and the outcome of such consultation.

Risk Management and Emergency Response Policies and Procedures

1. The medical fitness center must have a written emergency response plan that enables a timely and appropriate response to any emergency event that threatens the health and safety of facility users.

2. With physician oversight in place, a medical fitness center must have an appropriate number of automated external defibrillators (AEDs) that are easily accessible for use.

3. A medical fitness center with aquatic areas must have specific written emergency plans for each pool.

Programs and Services

1. A medical fitness center must have programs and services that address the needs and interests of its users.

2. A medical fitness center with aquatic facilities must have written policies and procedures specific to the programs and services that are to be offered in each aquatic area.

Professional Staffing

1. A medical fitness center must employ one or more professionals who hold degree(s), certification(s), and/or license(s) appropriate to each program offered and the populations served.

2. All staff must maintain a current certificate in automated external defibrillation (AED) and cardiopulmonary resuscitation (CPR) from a qualified certifying organization.

3. A medical fitness center must provide a variety of training and continuing education opportunities for staff, utilizing relationships with and expertise of physicians, other community healthcare professionals and/or experts, conferences, and distance learning programs that are approved for continuing education credits.

4. A medical fitness center must demonstrate that all staff maintain current certification(s) and/or license(s) by meeting the continuing education requirements for their specific certifying or licensing bodies.

Operational Policies and Practices

1. A medical fitness center must have a system in place that accurately monitors who has entered and remains in the facility at any given time.

2. A medical fitness center must have a system in place for helping ensure that every user achieves the maximum benefits of his or her exercise and program participation.

3. A medical fitness center must comply with all local, state, and federal laws and regulations governing the operation of the facility, including, but not limited to, building codes, the ADA, and OSHA requirements.

4. A medical fitness center with aquatic facilities must comply with all local and state laws and regulations regarding pool chemistry, chemical storage, pool supervision, signage, and so on.

5. A medical fitness center must meet all current local, state, and OSHA requirements for potentially hazardous materials, including handling of bodily fluids.

Signage

1. A medical fitness center must conspicuously post the appropriate signage, indicating caution, danger, and warning, in those locations that warrant such signage.

2. A medical fitness center must post all required ADA and OSHA signage.

3. A medical fitness center must post signage involving fire and related emergency situations as required by local, state, and federal regulations and codes.

Quality Management

1. A medical fitness center must have a systematic process in place to continuously assess and improve all aspects of health and fitness delivery, including, but not limited to, individual user outcomes, clinical and nonclinical programs and services, and operational and business processes.

Comparison of ACSM's Standards and the NSF Standard for Health/Fitness Facilities

For more than a year, two renowned organizations—the American College of Sports Medicine and NSF International—have simultaneously engaged in efforts to develop a set of standards for health/fitness facilities that are designed to ensure that the programs and activities members and users experience in a particular facility are both appropriate and safe. Given this, two key questions arise. First, why two separate sets of standards? And second, what differences exist between the two sets of standards? As the information in this appendix details, while ACSM's Standards and the NSF Standard are substantially the same, some differences exist, primarily because the two sets of standards target two distinctly dissimilar groups.

ACSM's Health/Fitness Facility Standards and Guidelines

The fourth edition of *ACSM's Health/Fitness Facility Standards and Guidelines* includes a total of 32 standards that specify base performance criteria (minimum requirements) that each health/fitness facility (staffed or unstaffed) must meet in order to satisfy its obligations to provide a reasonably safe and engaging physical activity environment for its members and users. Based on a consensus of ACSM and industry leaders, these standards are not intended to give rise to a legal duty of care. In addition to the 32 standards, this document includes a host of guidelines that represent recommendations that ACSM believes health/fitness operators should consider implementing to improve the overall quality of service they provide users. Such guidelines are not intended as standards, nor are they globally applicable; rather, they are intended as illustrative tools that health/fitness facility operators might consider.

NSF Standard

The efforts of NSF International, an American National Standards Institute (ANSI) accredited organization, under the leadership of the Joint Committee on Health Fitness Facilities, focused on development of its version of a voluntary Health/Fitness

Facility Standard following a process that complies with ANSI's requirements for transparency and due process. NSF International embarked on the development of its version of a Health/Fitness Standard in 2007. The NSF Standard is a result of a transparent process that involved a number of steps, including assessing previously published or documented health/fitness facility industry standards and guidelines, including the third edition of the *ACSM Health/Fitness Facility Standards and Guidelines*, the *Medical Fitness Association's Standards and Guidelines for Medical Fitness Facilities*, and *ASTM F1749 Standard Specification for Fitness Equipment and Health/Fitness Facility Safety Signage and Labels*. The NSF Standard has two key objectives: first, to provide a blueprint that specifies base performance criteria (minimum requirements) that the NSF Joint Committee and its various task groups believe that each *staffed* health/fitness facility must address to meet its obligations to provide a reasonably safe and engaging exercise environment for its members and users, and second, to become the foundation for a voluntary health/fitness facility certification process.

While the two sets of standards are closely aligned, both in their scope and language, a few differences exist. Unquestionably, the most significant difference relates to the target audience.

In the case of ACSM, its standards and guidelines are intended for a very broad audience (i.e., any and all health/fitness facilities, whether staffed or unstaffed, that provide services and programs to the general public). As for NSF, its standard is for a more narrowly defined audience (i.e., those facilities that are staffed during all operating hours). The accompanying table provides a comparison of ACSM's Standards as they appear in the fourth edition and the NSF Standard, which is progressing through the development and approval process.

Table L.1

In the accompanying table that highlights the primary differences that exist between the two sets of standards, in the numerical designator, the first number refers to the number of the standard as it appears in a particular set of standards. The second number identifies a subset of that specific standard.

Due to the proprietary nature of the NSF Standard, providing specific wording for each of the approved standards is not feasible. Instead, the NSF Standard is identified in table L.1 by the number (refer to explanation in previous paragraph) that most closely aligns with the corresponding ACSM Standard. In addition, the perceived intent underlying each of the NSF Standards is noted.

TABLE L.1	Comparison of ACSM's Health/Fitness Facility Standards and the NSF Standard for Health/Fitness Facilities	
ACSM's Standards, fourth edition	**Similar NSF Standard**	**Intent of the NSF Standard**
1.1 Facility operators shall offer a general pre-activity screening tool (e.g., Par-Q) and/or specific pre-activity screening tool (e.g., health risk appraisal [HRA], health history questionnaire [HHQ]) to all new members and prospective users.	2.1 and 2.1.1	To ensure that all health/fitness facilities offer a form or pre-activity screening tool to all new members and users and that, furthermore, when members or users fail to participate in a pre-activity screening, they are required to acknowledge their decision in writing.
1.2 General pre-activity screening tools (e.g., Par-Q) shall provide an authenticated means for new members, and/or users to identify whether a level of risk exists that indicates that they should seek consultation from a qualified healthcare professional prior to engaging in a program of physical activity.	2.2	To ensure that any general or simple pre-activity screening tool provides a means by which members/users can identify their level of risk and, furthermore, that the pre-activity screening tool provides them with guidance on seeking appropriate professional advice before embarking on an exercise program.
1.3 All specific pre-activity screening tools (e.g., HRA, HHQ) shall be reviewed and interpreted by qualified staff (e.g., a qualified health/fitness professional or healthcare professional), and the results of the review and interpretation shall be retained on file by the facility for a period of at least one year from the time the tool was reviewed and interpreted.	2.3	To ensure that any detailed pre-activity screening tool, such as a health history questionnaire, is reviewed and assessed by a qualified health/fitness professional. Furthermore, if individuals are found to have a disease or composite of risk factors that pose an increased risk to them if they begin exercising, they are advised to seek the appropriate consultation from a healthcare provider before beginning their exercise program.

ACSM's Standards, fourth edition	Similar NSF Standard	Intent of the NSF Standard
1.4 If a facility operator becomes aware that a member, user, or prospective user has a known cardiovascular, metabolic, or pulmonary disease, or two or more major cardiovascular risk factors, or any self-disclosed medical concern, that individual shall be advised to consult with a qualified healthcare provider before beginning a physical activity program.	2.3	Same as previous.
1.5 Facilities shall provide a means for communicating to existing members (e.g., those who have been members for greater than 90 days) the value of completing a general and/or specific pre-activity screening tool on a regular basis (e.g., preferably once annually) during the course of their membership. Such communication can be done through a variety of mechanisms, including but not limited to a statement incorporated into the membership agreement of the facility, a statement on the new-member pre-activity screening form, and a statement on the website.	2.4	To ensure that health/fitness facility operators communicate to individuals the importance of participating in a pre-activity screening protocol on a regular basis in order to allow appropriate facility personnel to become aware of any possible changes in their health status.
2.1 Once a new member or prospective user has completed a pre-activity screening process, facility operators shall then offer the new member or prospective user a general orientation to the facility.	3.1	To ensure that health/fitness facility members and users are offered some form of orientation process that allows them to receive the proper guidance in embarking on an exercise program.
2.2 Facilities shall provide a means by which members and users who are engaged in a physical activity program within the facility can obtain assistance and/or guidance with their physical activity program.	3.2	To ensure that once a member or user has embarked on an exercise program that the facility operator provides a means by which that individual can obtain guidance or assistance with their activity program.
3.1 Facility operators must have written emergency response policies and procedures, which shall be reviewed regularly and physically rehearsed at least twice annually. These policies shall enable staff to respond to basic first-aid situations and emergency events in an appropriate and timely manner.	4.1.1	To ensure that health/fitness facility operators have in place an emergency response system and, furthermore, that all employees of the facility are trained in basic CPR/AED administration as well as in the facility's emergency response system.
3.2 Facility operators shall ensure that a safety audit is conducted that routinely inspects all areas of the facility to reduce or eliminate unsafe hazards that may cause injury to employees and health/fitness facility members or health/fitness facility users.	4.1.2	To ensure that facility operators incorporate some form of safety inspection process that will assist in reducing potential safety hazards.
3.3 Facility operators shall have a written system for sharing information with members and users, employees, and independent contractors regarding the handling of potentially hazardous materials, including the handling of bodily fluids by the facility staff in accordance with the guidelines of the U.S. Occupational Safety and Health Administration (OSHA).	4.2	To ensure that facility operators provide information to members and users as well as staff regarding handling hazardous materials and materials that may contain bloodborne pathogens.
3.4 In addition to complying with all applicable federal, state, and local requirements relating to automated external defibrillators (AEDs), all facilities (i.e., staffed and unstaffed) shall have as part of their written emergency response policies and procedures a public access defibrillation (PAD) program in accordance with general accepted practice, as highlighted in this section.	4.3, 4.3.2, 4.3.3, 4.3.4, 4.3.5, 4.3.6	To ensure that facility operators comply with all applicable federal, state, and local laws regarding public access defibrillation (PAD) in the facility setting, and that even in the absence of any formal laws that facility operators have as part of their emergency response systems a PAD program that meets with the generally accepted practices of a PAD program.
3.5 AEDs in a facility shall be located within a 1.5-minute walk to any place an AED could be potentially needed.	4.3.1	To ensure that AEDs are properly placed in the facility so that they are placed within a 3-minute response time of any potential cardiac-related event.
3.6 A skills review, practice sessions, and a practice drill with the AED shall be conducted a minimum of every six months, covering a variety of potential emergency situations (e.g., water, presence of a pacemaker, medications, children).	4.1.1	To ensure that facility operators have a plan in place involving procedures for regularly rehearsing their emergency response system and that all new staff are appropriately trained in the facility's procedures as soon as reasonably possible after they are hired.

(continued)

ACSM's Standards, fourth edition	Similar NSF Standard	Intent of the NSF Standard
3.7 A staffed facility shall assign at least one staff member to be on duty during all facility operating hours who is currently trained and certified in the delivery of cardiopulmonary resuscitation and in the administration of an AED.	4.3.6	To ensure that a facility has at least one staff member on duty during operating hours who is presently trained and certified in the administration of CPR and an AED.
3.8 Unstaffed facilities must comply with all applicable federal, state, and local requirements relating to AEDs. Unstaffed facilities shall have as part of their written emergency response policies and procedures a PAD program as a means by which either members and users or an external emergency responder can respond from time of collapse to defibrillation in four minutes or less.	None applicable.	
4.1 The health/fitness professionals who have supervisory responsibility and oversight responsibility for the physical activity programs and the staff who administer them shall have an appropriate level of professional education, work experience, and/or certification. Examples of health/fitness professionals who serve in a supervisory role include the fitness director, group exercise director, aquatics director, and program director.	5.1	To ensure that the supervisory staff responsible for the facility's physical activity programs have the proper level of competency as evidenced by their level of experience, education, and/or certification.
4.2 The health/fitness and healthcare professionals who serve in counseling, instruction, and physical activity supervision roles for the facility shall have an appropriate level of professional education, work experience, and/or certification. The primary professional staff and independent contractors who serve in these roles are fitness instructors, group exercise instructors, lifestyle counselors, and personal trainers.	5.2	To ensure that the fitness professionals responsible for providing exercise coaching, exercise instruction, and exercise supervision for the facility's members and users have the proper level of competency as evidenced by their level of experience, education, and/or certification.
4.3 Health/fitness and healthcare professionals engaged in pre-activity screening or prescribing, instructing, monitoring, or supervising of physical activity programs for facility members and users shall have current automated external defibrillation and cardiopulmonary resuscitation (AED and CPR) certification from an organization qualified to provide such certification. A certification should include a practical examination.	5.3	To ensure that all fitness professionals involved in activities involving coaching, instructing, prescribing, or supervising members and users in exercise are currently certified in the administration of CPR and an AED.
5.1 Facilities shall have an operational system in place that monitors, either manually or technologically, the presence and identity of all individuals (e.g., members and users) who enter into and participate in the activities, programs, and services of the facility.	7.2	To ensure that facility operators have in place protocols for monitoring the presence and identity of all individuals who enter their facility and that, furthermore, the facility operator has a protocol for verifying that no individual remains in the facility after the facility has closed for the day.
5.2 Facilities that offer a sauna, steam room, or whirlpool shall have a technical monitoring system in place to ensure that these areas are maintained at the proper temperature and humidity level and that the appropriate warning systems and signage are in place to notify members and users of any risks related to the use of these areas, including subsequent unsafe changes in temperature and humidity.	7.3	To ensure that health/fitness facilities that offer wet or thermal amenities, such as saunas, maintain those areas at recognized safe environmental levels and that the proper signage is posted alerting individuals to the potential risks inherent in using these amenities.
5.3 Facilities that offer members and users access to a pool or whirlpool shall provide evidence that they comply with all water-chemistry safety requirements mandated by state and local codes and regulations.	7.4	To ensure that health/fitness facilities that offer aquatic amenities and environments, such as pools, provide evidence that they operate those environments in accordance with all legally mandated regulations.
5.4 A facility that offers youth services or programs shall provide evidence that it complies with all applicable state and local laws and regulations pertaining to their supervision.	7.5	To ensure that facility operators that offer programs and services for youth comply with all legally mandated regulations regarding supervision of these programs and services.

ACSM's Standards, fourth edition	Similar NSF Standard	Intent of the NSF Standard
5.5 When a child is under direct staff supervision of a facility, as a participant in either an organized activity or in an ongoing facility program, or is just under temporary staff supervision while the parent or legal guardian is using the facility, the responsible staff person shall have ready access to the child's basic medical information, which has been previously collected from the parent as part of the child registration process.	7.5.1	To ensure that a designated facility operator has the appropriate medical and/or health information on all youth left under their supervision.
5.6 The registration policy of a facility that provides child care shall require that parents or guardians of all children left in the facility's care complete a waiver, an authorization for emergency medical care, and a release for the children whom they leave under the temporary care of the facility.	7.5.2	To ensure that parents and/or legal guardians of youth left under the supervision of the facility operator have provided written authorization pertaining to emergency medical care for their youth.
5.7 The facility shall require that parents and guardians provide the facility with names of persons who are authorized by the parent or legal guardian to pick up each child. The facility shall not release children to any unauthorized person, and furthermore, the facility shall maintain records of the date and time each child checked out and was dropped off and the name of the person to whom the child was released.	7.5.3	To ensure that a designated facility operator receives from parents or legal guardians the names of any individual authorized to pick up their children and that, furthermore, the facility operator maintains an accurate record of when children are left under their supervision and/or removed from under their supervision.
5.8 Facilities shall have written policies regarding children's issues, such as requirements for staff providing supervision of children, age limits for children, restroom practices, food, and parental presence on site. Facilities shall inform parents and guardians of these policies and require that parents and guardians sign a form that acknowledges that they have received the policies, understand the policies, and will abide by the policies.	7.5.4	To ensure that health/fitness facility operators have written policies pertaining to their youth programs and services.
None applicable.	7.5.5	To ensure that facility operators perform criminal-background checks on any staff who are responsible for the supervision of children under the direct responsibility of the facility.
6.1 Facilities, to the extent required by law, must adhere to the standards of building design that relate to the designing, building, expanding, or renovating of space as detailed in the Americans with Disabilities Act (ADA).	6.3	To ensure that health/fitness facilities comply with all applicable ADA laws and regulations.
6.2 Facilities must be in compliance with all federal, state, and local building codes.	6	To ensure that all health/fitness facilities are in compliance with all legally mandated building and occupancy codes.
7.1 The aquatic and pool facilities must provide the proper safety equipment according to state and local codes and regulations.	6.2	To ensure that all health/fitness facilities are in compliance with all legally mandated laws and regulations pertaining to equipment and signage in the facility.
8.1 Facility operators shall post proper caution, danger, and warning signage in conspicuous locations where facility staff know, or should know, that existing conditions and situations warrant such signage.	8.1	To ensure that facility operators provide the proper cautionary, warning, and danger signage in their facility when conditions exist that warrant the placement of such signage and that the signage comply with all legally mandated laws and regulations.
8.2 Facility operators shall post the appropriate emergency and safety signage pertaining to fire and related emergency situations, as required by federal, state, and local codes.	8.2, 8.2.1, 8.2.2, 8.2.4	To ensure that the facility has the proper legally mandated signage pertaining to emergency situations, such as fire emergencies.
8.3 Facility operators shall post signage indicating the location of any AED and first-aid kits, including directions on how to access those locations.	8.2.3	To ensure that facility operators provide signage that clearly identifies the location of and directions to first aid and AED equipment.

(continued)

TABLE L.1, *continued*

ACSM's Standards, fourth edition	Similar NSF Standard	Intent of the NSF Standard
8.4 Facilities shall post all ADA and OSHA signage that is required by federal, state, and local laws and regulations.	8.3	To ensure that all legally mandated signage pertaining to ADA and OSHA is properly posted in the facility.
8.5 All cautionary, danger, and warning signage shall have the required signal icon, signal word, signal color, and layout as specified in ASTM F1749.	8.4	To ensure that when conditions exist that could endanger members or users that the facility post the proper cautionary, warning, and danger signage and that this signage adhere to the guidelines set forth by ASTM Standard F1749.

Bibliography

American College of Sports Medicine. *ACSM's guidelines for exercise testing and prescription. 7th Edition.* Philadelphia: Lippincott, Williams and Wilkins; 2006.

American College of Sports Medicine. *ACSM's health and fitness facility standards and guidelines. 2nd Edition.* Champaign, IL: Human Kinetics; 1997.

American College of Sports Medicine. *ACSM's resource manual for guidelines for exercise testing and prescription. 5th Edition.* Philadelphia: Lippincott, Williams and Wilkins; 2006.

American College of Sports Medicine and American Heart Association. *Joint position statement on automated external defibrillators in health/fitness facilities.* 2002.

American Heart Association and American College of Sports Medicine. *Joint statement: Recommendations for cardiovascular screening, staffing and emergency policies at health/fitness facilities. Circulation* 30(6): 1-19. 1998.

American Heart Association. *Guidelines for cardiopulmonary resuscitation and emergency cardiovascular care 2010.* 2010.

Grantham, W.C.; Patton, R.W.; York, T.D.; Winick, M.L. *Health fitness management.* Champaign, IL: Human Kinetics; 1998.

Herbert, D.L.; Herbert, W.G. *Legal aspects of preventive, rehabilitative and recreational exercise programs. 4th Edition.* Canton, OH: PRC Publishing; 2002.

International Health, Racquet and Sportsclub Association. *Health and safety, legal and ethical standards for U.S. IHRSA clubs: Standards facilitation guide.* Boston: 1998.

International Health, Racquet and Sportsclub Association. *IHRSA. Global report: State of the health club industry.* Boston: 2002, 2003, 2004, and 2005.

International Health, Racquet and Sportsclub Association. *IHRSA's 2010 profiles of success.* Boston: 2010.

Tharrett, S. *Fitness management. 2nd Edition.* Monterey, CA: Healthy Learning; 2008.

United States Access Board. *Accessible sports facilities: A summary of accessibility guidelines for recreation facilities.* Supplement to Americans with Disabilities Act Access Guidelines. 2002.

United States Access Board. *Accessible swimming pools and spas: A summary of accessibility guidelines for recreation facilities.* Supplement to Americans with Disabilities Act Access Guidelines. 2002.

Index

Note: The italicized *f* and *t* following page numbers refer to figures and tables, respectively.